WHEN BAD BACKS HAPPEN TO GOOD PEOPLE

WHEN BAD BACKS HAPPEN TO GOOD PEOPLE

IT'S NOT ALL IN YOUR HEAD

Jordan S. Fersel, MD

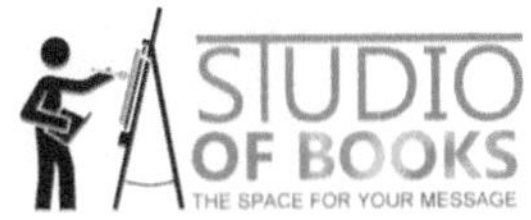

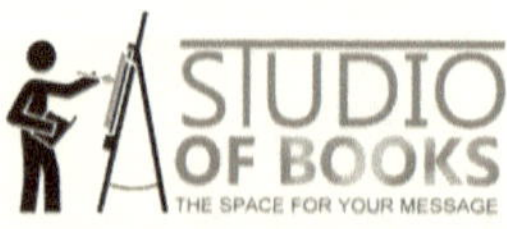

Studio of Books LLC
5900 Balcones Drive Suite 100
Austin, Texas 78731
www.studioofbooks.org
Hotline: (254) 800-1183

Ordering Information:
Special discounts are available on quantity purchases by corporations, associations, and others. For details, contact the publisher at the address above.

Printed in the United States of America.

ISBN-13:   Softcover: 978-1-968491-58-1

            eBook: 978-1-968491-59-8

Library of Congress Control Number: 2025917158

"Failing to deal with physical causes of pain will not allow for complete psychological healing and vice versa."

This book primarily focuses on chronic pain affecting the back and neck, but it also explores a range of other topics. These include medical concerns, spinal architecture, facet issues, sacroiliac joint problems, nerve complexities, arthritis, treatments, and healing processes. Written by a physician trained in pain management, the text focuses on the goals of decreasing pain and stress while increasing activity, sleep, and sociability. It explores the difference between acute and chronic pain, the statistics regarding back pain and chronic pain, and then examines the spinal and nervous system, including the facet and sacroiliac joints.

Fersel also explores the aging population and arthritis, highlighting the importance of a healthy lifestyle, and then focuses on treatment options, with surgery reserved as a last resort. Other options discussed include narcotic medicine (along with its pros and cons), meditation, using a TENS unit, breathing exercises, yoga, chiropractic treatment, physical therapy, swimming, stretching, acupuncture, massage, and the use of a spinal cord stimulator. The author's book focuses on chronic pain as a symptom, not an illness. Ultimately, it offers hope for the patient's future.

The book effectively conveys complex issues in a readable manner, focusing on chronic pain as a medical condition and not as an illness. Using personal and professional stories as well as case studies makes the text more relatable to the reader. It is a hopeful text that supports the patient. The drawings/diagrams are excellent, although the photos are not of the same quality. At times, the book employs certain medical terms that may be unfamiliar to the average reader. However, overall, this is a helpful text and suitable for those seeking a beginner's book on chronic back pain.

*Reviewed by **Carol Anderson, D.Min., ACSW, MSW**, The US Review of Books*
Professional Review for the People

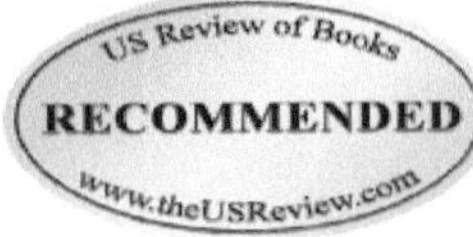

Acknowledgements

To Esty,

Without your encouragement, this book would exist only in my mind.

Medical Illustrations:
Laurie O'Keefe

Cover design:
Arielle Leventhal

Much gratitude to my friend, Howard Druce, M.D. for reviewing the manuscript and providing many insightful thoughts and ideas.

Table *of* Contents

"I was sitting writing at my textbook but the work did not progress; my thoughts were elsewhere. I turned my chair to the fire and dozed. Again the atoms were gamboling before my eyes. This time the smaller groups kept modestly in the background. My mental eye, rendered more acute by the repeated visions of the kind could now distinguish larger structures of manifold conformation; long rows, sometimes more closely fitted together all twining and twisting in snake like motion. But look! What was that? One of the snakes had seized hold of its own tail, and the form whirled mockingly before my eyes (Figure 1).

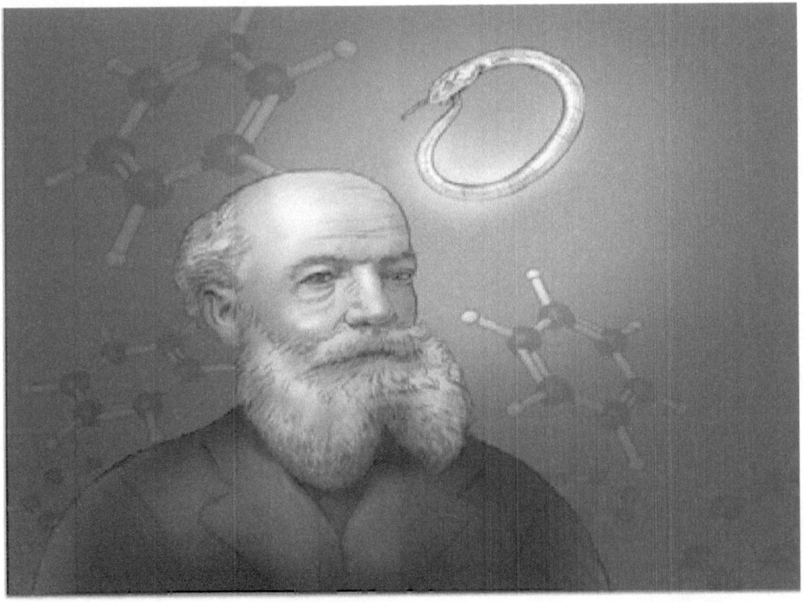

Figure 1. August Kekule, discoverer of circular benzene ring.

"As if by a flash of lightning I awoke; and this time also I spent the rest of the night in working out the rest of the hypothesis. Let us learn to dream, gentleman, then perhaps we shall find the truth...But let us beware of publishing our dreams till they have been tested by waking understanding."[1]

---

1   August Kekule at Benzolfest In Berichte 23 (1890), 1302.

Introduction

This is a book about observation, imagination, philosophy, and filling in the missing gaps of information in order to help you better understand and deal with your chronic pain. If you have purchased this book, you are likely not satisfied with the ways in which your suffering has been viewed and treated by the medical establishment. You may have tried many, if not most, remedies, read many books on the topic of neck/back pain, and have alternately been excited and disappointed by new treatments and cures found on the Internet. I understand that you are going through a difficult period in your life, that your relationships may be at risk, and that frustration follows you like a dark cloud. I am totally sympathetic to what you are experiencing, and I would like you to understand from a systematic, mechanistic approach what is happening to you and what can be done to decrease your pain and suffering.

What qualifications do I have to write this book?

I am a board-certified fellowship trained physician. Those certifications by themselves do not qualify me as a world-class expert in treating chronic pain; there are many other specialists who have similar training and experience. A doctor, in the course of his or her career, makes many observations. An innovator in the field of medicine distills these observations into meaningful patterns and then, rules. I have made more than ten thousand patient observations from conducting second opinions, also known as independent medical evaluations (IMEs). In the process of performing these IMEs, I have had the opportunity to review the questions asked by other treating physicians and their physical examinations and interpretation of objective data such as x-rays and MRI scans and diagnoses and treatment plans. From this experience, I have been able to piece together what happens to the spine in cases of illness, injury, and trauma.

The scientific method of observation is denigrated in our more enlightened age of computer-assisted diagnosis. I am fortunate to have had the experience of informally collecting large amounts of data and observing which tests, therapies, and treatments are useful and which ones are not. I believe that my experience is unique and allows for a very different perspective from most clinicians and academics. The focus in recent times has been on randomized clinical trials, and while that is certainly the gold standard for investigation and research, in practice it becomes difficult to apply in humans who will suffer in this process of randomization, from the introduction of placebos and sham procedures. In addition, before we subject humans to clinical trials, we should focus in a laser-fine way on the problem we wish to investigate. We owe this to our patients who may also be our research subjects.

Since there are so many potential causes of low back pain, it would make a great deal of sense to have some idea of how to classify the different causes for pain and also have some idea of the way that they occur (mechanism) and of the frequency of their occurrence (epidemiology). These approaches are rarely taken and are out of necessity observational in nature. Some of science and technology today is about finding solutions to problems that do not or only rarely do exist. Chronic pain and especially low back pain is pervasive in our society and a function of the way we have chosen to live, work, and exercise, to eat and to play. Our lifestyle choices are very important and should be the starting point for any meaningful scientific inquiry.

Why did I choose to title this book It's Not All in Your Head?

Certain physicians have been very successful in helping many people control and diminish their complaints of low back pain. One thesis has been that many individuals can have gastrointestinal distress or low back pain as a result of psychological stress. Individuals can have different areas in the body that are sensitive to stress. In the case of low back pain, the muscle spasm that occurs can persist unless interrupted by patients becoming aware of those issues in their subconscious mind that are upsetting, thus defeating the mind's strategy to repress these emotions. It is thought that by using these strategies the back pain becomes purposeless and fades away. This approach has been very successful, and many people swear by it. I agree with the concept of the mind-body connection, and one can certainly not argue with the results, but no one has ever demonstrated a cause-and-effect relationship between the repression of thoughts and feelings in the subconscious mind and chronic low back pain. It is clear though that the mind has a powerful influence on the nervous system and consequently the relaxation of muscles.

Let's say that you have attempted to treat your back pain with mind-body or other psychological methods, and you continue to suffer from low back pain. What is happening? There are two possibilities. Either you have failed to apply these principles properly and you should continue your efforts to relax your subconscious mind, or the pain is of an anatomic, physical basis, and the reason that mind-body methods are not helpful is that the problem resides somewhere other than the subconscious mind. It is highly unlikely that every patient suffering from chronic low back pain has issues of repression in their subconscious mind. There are definitely identifiable physical causes for chronic pain in some patients, even if there are also psychological factors at play. Failing to deal with physical causes of pain will not allow for complete psychological healing and vice versa.

For patients who have tried mind-body techniques and continue to suffer, this book will provide additional valuable information and possible therapeutic options.

Why did I find it necessary to write this book?

Over the years, I have observed many patients who were desperate to relieve their chronic pain. Many of these patients have turned to surgical intervention in an effort to relieve or diminish their pain. This is a completely rational response, and if low back surgery had better results, it would be a logical conclusion. Unfortunately, in many cases the results are not favorable, and the patient may continue with the same, or even new, pain following surgery. I have tried to encourage patients to avoid low back surgery whenever feasible. Obviously, patients must have other options that help them in order for them to accept and heed my warnings. Alternatives to surgery are discussed in this book, but my true focus will be to teach you about the real reasons for your chronic pain—reasons that are in harmony with an understanding of the structure and function of your body.

What methods have I used other than observation to form my conclusions?

The backbone (pardon the pun) of this work is the observations from thousands of patient contacts along with the ability to learn from patient reports which treatments have and have not been helpful. It is not a reasonable goal to totally eradicate chronic pain for any individual patient, but certainly for most patients, chronic pain can be diminished. Decreasing pain allows patients to sleep better, increase activity levels, interact socially with others without the distraction or frustration of pain, and diminish the stress response and raised cortisol levels.

In order to bring about these types of changes in a complex system, such as the pain-sensing system in the body, it is useful to employ concepts of reverse engineering and systems biology. Reverse engineering is taking apart an object to see how it works in order to duplicate or enhance the object.[2] If a U.S. drone is shot down over China and the drone is taken apart and studied and the result is the blueprint for the manufacturing of similar drones by China, this is an example of reverse engineering. In genetics, similar results have been achieved by manipulating the genome to manufacture specific proteins. This is an example of systems biology in which "systems of biological components, which may be molecules, cells, tissues, organisms, or entire species are studied." Living tissues are dynamic and complex and are best understood in the context of their role within a system, such as the role of nerves within the nervous system

---

2   Reverse engineering definition: WhatIs.com, Margaret Rouse.

and the propagation of chronic pain. Tissue "behavior may be hard to predict from the properties of the individual parts."[3]

I have been able to observe which descriptions of pain, which signs on physical examination, and which objective findings, such as MRI and EMG results, are most significant in terms of deciding the best practices for diagnosis and treatment, in my opinion. Think of restoring a shattered mirror or piece of pottery. It is unlikely that we will have all the pieces, but our objective generally is to get the best fit. On every level, this has been my goal to discover the optimal interpretation of subjective complaints, objective findings on physical exam and radiologic and nerve testing, while giving consideration to the unique features of human anatomy and physiology, especially as it relates to the upright posture of human beings, and to explain what this means to you.

The nervous system is the most complex system of the human body. One of its many functions is the sensation of pain. There are many other functions of the nervous system, such as memory, cognition, learning, emotion, position sense, locomotion, fight- or-flight response, and special senses such as sight, hearing, taste, and smell. This list is by no means exhaustive, and new abilities and properties of the nervous system are constantly being discovered. Recently an anatomic connection between the nervous and immune systems was discovered. I cannot promise that my explanation of chronic neck/back pain will alleviate your pain, but if I have given you a new perspective for understanding and treating your pain and suffering, and have in general way discouraged you from undergoing unnecessary low back/neck surgery, together we have accomplished a great deal. I also cannot promise that everyone will be helped, because some types of chronic pain are more complex, are poorly understood, require additional study, and may be challenging to treat.

This book is not meant to be a comprehensive medical textbook for the treatment of chronic low back pain. It is rather a guide that patients can use in order to get the greatest benefit from their treatments with

---

3   Systems biology definition: sysbio.med.Harvard.edu.

minimum delay. Health care professionals can read this book for a new perspective that may differ from that presented in their formal medical education. I hope that if you are living with chronic pain that you will be able to use the information in these pages to ease your pain and suffering.

Chapter 1

Chronic Pain

Understanding the Problem

All doctors are taught in medical school that the most common reason that patients seek office visits is due to pain. Most of these complaints are of a short-term, acute basis for reasons such as appendicitis, kidney stones or gallstones, or bone, muscle, or joint injuries. In some cases, the acute pain is a harbinger of something more serious, such as chest or jaw pain indicating blockage of a coronary artery, or mid to upper back pain that may precede rupture of an aortic aneurysm. In all these cases, the pain that occurs is a useful signal, in the sense that it brings the patient to the doctor to seek treatment and it gives the physician valuable clues as to what is ailing the patient and the manner in which corrective action should be pursued. We are fortunate to have such a mechanism associated with our consciousness, as the acute component of pain almost always serves as a valuable early warning system.

Interestingly, the converse is not true. There are many disease conditions that do not cause pain or even present with painful symptoms. Even in the case of cancer, possibly due to the type, size, location, and rate of growth of the lesion, the presenting symptoms do not always include pain. Our pain system is not without its deficiencies. In fact, severe chest pain, which mimics a heart attack, can be caused by esophageal reflux or inflammation of joints along the anterior (front) chest wall. The acute pain warning system is not always specific and usually requires analysis by a trained professional to help sort out the possibilities (diagnosis) and to put together an action plan (treatment).

In an ideal world, all pain would have meaning, point to a specific cause for the pain (or at least help narrow down the list of possibilities), motivate the patient to seek help within a reasonable amount of time, and cease to send out painful messages once the problem has been resolved. As a general rule, this is true of acute pain.

If there is an abscess, drainage and antibiotics will usually resolve both the infection and pain. For fractures, setting and immobilizing broken bones will dampen the pain message as healing begins, and for a surgical problem like appendicitis, as I am sure you know, an appendectomy to remove the source of infection and inflammation. At any stage of healing from any acute problem, there can be complications or new reasons for pain. If the infection is resistant to antibiotics, or there was an area of the bone that did not heal properly, or any one of a number of scenarios, you can be certain that the patient will experience additional pain. This acute pain is an indication that healing is not proceeding in a normal or orderly fashion. It is not much fun to have a complication, but we can agree that the pain is still useful in terms of the information it provides. As problems get resolved, healing can go forward, and acute pain recedes. It is apparent that acute pain, inflammation, and healing form the basis for the body's detection that something is amiss and for the initiation of the repair process.

I find it useful to think of acute pain as the check-engine light on your car's dashboard. When the indicator lights up, there is usually an issue to be attended to. Ignore the warning and be prepared to spend a lot of money fixing something that at the outset was in many cases relatively easy to manage.

Chronic pain, on the other hand, is a thorny issue. It is all encompassing in the sense that it can take over a person's life—not only the physical features but also the psychological, emotional, and physiological (the way that the organ systems work) aspects. (See figure 2.)

In addition, society grapples with such issues as inadequate pain control, issues of suicide, death and dying, and the troubling issues of addiction and overdose, including problems emanating from abuse, misuse, and over prescription of narcotic analgesics. This does not even begin to address the actual costs to society of caring for and treating the chronic pain population.

ACUTE PAIN	CHRONIC PAIN
...is caused by external or internal injury or damage.	...is uncoupled from the causative event.
...has an intensity that correlates with the triggering stimulus.	...has an intensity that no longer correlates with the triggering stimulus.
...can be clearly located.	...becomes a disease in its own right.
...has distinct warning and protective functions.	...has lost its warning and protective functions.
	...is a special therapeutic challenge.

Figure 2. Acute versus chronic pain.

It should be clear that chronic pain has personal, interpersonal, familial, communal, political, and societal aspects. There are very few problems in life that approach this level of complexity. People have divergent and polarizing opinions on this matter. Several years ago, a retired recovery room nurse who I knew well, made an appointment to see me in my office. This was no ordinary appointment. She proceeded to explain to me that her son who had chronic shoulder pain, had recently died of an overdose of narcotics prescribed for him by his medical doctor. At that point, I could only listen to her and share her grief. She was adamant that patients like her son not be treated with narcotics beyond the phase of acute pain. I could understand her point, but I do not necessarily agree. I am certain that there are many family members, friends, and coworkers who have witnessed the devastation caused by narcotic analgesics used improperly who would agree. In this book, I will stress how essential it is for patients to have a proper diagnosis so that they do not receive excessive amounts of pain medications. Some patients, despite our efforts to limit their exposure to narcotics, will still require pain medications in order to be functional. I will discuss this issue more fully in Chapter 10.

I will attempt to clarify some of these issues and try to get a sharper focus on diagnosis and treatment of one type of chronic pain, low back pain.

In order to understand the effects of chronic pain, we must better define it. Twenty-five years ago, the climate in the specialty of pain management was very different; very few people were sympathetic to the problems of chronic pain patients. In fact, due to the doctor's inability to produce a cure in many cases, patients were labeled as having personality disorders or neuroses. If I have pain from my gallbladder and my physician incorrectly diagnosed esophageal reflux, does that make me neurotic or mentally ill? Of course not! There have also been some notable cases where depression is responsible for the exacerbation or even the cause of pain, but they are not common. At the time, doctors were suspicious of patients in terms of their motives, and the patients, those truly experiencing chronic pain, regarded their doctors as arrogant and ineffective. Hopefully as we get a better understanding of chronic pain, these attitudes will evolve.

The International Association for the Study of Pain (IASP) defines chronic pain as pain that persists beyond the time that normal healing takes place, typically from three to six months.[4] There are a number of other characteristics associated with chronic pain not found in acute pain. I think that a better definition of chronic pain is - pain that represents an abnormal physiologic response, brought on by damage to a part of the nervous system, which results in prolonged or unbroken periods of pain and suffering. Some have suggested that chronic pain can be unresponsive to treatment, but this statement is not universally true.

The fact that most clinicians miss is that it is *damaged or overstimulated nerve tissue* that is responsible for pain. An inflamed or infected nerve will let out a "scream" that is sometimes indescribable. When you have a toothache, it is not the tooth that is feeling the pain but rather the specialized nerve apparatus inside the tooth that is sensing pain and transmitting that sensation. This results in *the experience* of pain, with its interpretation as suffering in the brain. When the dentist sprays your cavity with air or water, don't you just want to hit the ceiling? The air or water is brushing by the exposed nerve that the dentist has exposed by removing decay. In a similar fashion, pain from kidney stones or gallstones is not from the stones themselves but from the hyper-stimulation of the specialized nerves within smooth muscle, which transmit the rhythmic spasmodic sensations of the ureter or gallbladder contracting, first to your spine and then to the brain. There are fine nerves located throughout the body on the surface of bones and within joints and muscles that sense and monitor for tissue damage. Of course, the largest organ in your body, the skin, is chock-full of sensory nerves because this is where we do most of our interfacing with the external environment.

What happens when something goes awry with any of these sensory nerves? In much the same way that it is annoying and unsettling when your car or home alarm goes off, imagine how much worse it would be if no one could figure out how to turn the sound off. That is just a small taste of the way chronic pain is experienced by its sufferers. And people

---

4   IASP Classification of Chronic Pain —Pain 1986: Suppl. 3:S1-S226.

do suffer in their relationships, their jobs, their ability to remember things and to concentrate, and their ability to enjoy life. Suffering is the cognitive and emotional component of chronic pain that cannot easily be turned off. That is in addition to the fairly steady grind of the pain that is *always* present in some fashion.

Understanding the differences between acute and chronic pain is only the beginning of your healing. Obviously, in medicine, you the patient have to be able to describe the problem in order for the doctor to have a clue of how to help you ... but when this information makes its way to your doctor's esteemed cranium, something interesting happens, and it doesn't really have much to do with you, so if results are suboptimal and you are not satisfied, don't take it personally.

In this chapter, you have learned the following:

- the differences between acute and chronic pain, central and peripheral pain

- that chronic pain is, in essence, a disease of either damaged or chronically stimulated nerves, whether located in the central or peripheral nervous system, and may or may not be associated with frank tissue damage

Chapter 2

Medicine by the Numbers

The Challenge of Medical Decision Making

This is a true story. In my second year of medical school, just as we were learning about diseases of the kidney, I had my first kidney stone. I was in a lot of pain. I went to the student health services and was sent to Dr. G., a urologist, who coincidentally had been lecturing us about diseases of the kidneys. He did a diagnostic test in his office and told me that the stone would soon pass. I asked him what could have caused the kidney stone, and his demeanor changed. "Didn't you listen to my lecture on kidney stones?" he asked with impatience. I responded that we were having that lecture next week. "Oh," he said without missing a beat. "Well, make sure you show up." It was at that moment in my budding medical career that I decided that everyone, regardless of educational level, deserves an explanation from their doctor and not a lecture. By the way, I am still not sure what causes kidney stones exactly, but I sure know firsthand how much they hurt.

Why should you care about my story?

First, you must realize that no two doctors practice medicine in the same way. This is particularly true in the specialty of pain management where there is so much disputed information and so many ways to interpret diagnostic tests. Due to the fuzzy nature of chronic pain, there are numerous schools of thought with respect to causation of pain and its proper treatment. Second, every specialist performs consistent with the manner that he or she has been trained. I always tell patients, "If you want back surgery, go see a spine surgeon first." You know the old adage, "If your only tool is a hammer, then the whole world will seem like a nail." The same is true if you see any specialist; he or she will focus on their own areas of training and expertise. Third, we all have different personalities and biases that impact the ways that we relate to others. This is especially true when we are formulating first impressions of others (as in an initial consultation). Pain management is also a specialty that requires the clinician to evaluate both subjective complaints and objective findings in the context of a hostile and sometimes unreasonable insurance and regulatory environment.

Epidemiology is the study and analysis of the patterns, causes, and effects of health and disease conditions in defined populations. One of the most important roles of modern medicine had been to describe the incidence and prevalence of medical conditions. Incidence is defined as the number of times a disease or condition occurs in a population in the course of a year, and prevalence is the amount of times the condition is found within a population within a life span. What are your chances of experiencing low back or neck pain in your lifetime, from any cause?

Here are some of the most important statistics and scientific studies with respect to low back pain and how I choose to interpret this information. Up to 80 percent of us experience low back or neck pain in the course of our lives.[5] The problem with this statistic is that we mostly experience episodes of back or neck pain from muscle spasm or strain, or mild hyperextension of joints of the spine, which are usually self-limited and of brief duration, perceived mostly as acute pain. As far as I know, there are no large epidemiological studies of *chronic* neck and low back pain, but making an educated guess, the prevalence is no more than 10–15 percent, still a very large number of people, at any time.[6]

---

5   Low Back Pain Fact Sheet, www.ninds.nih.gov.
6   Family Practice 16 (1999): 475–482.

These concepts are important because in order to treat a condition, first we must understand how it develops. Most studies lump all patients together with a nonspecific diagnosis, such as chronic low back pain, but that does not help the clinician to evaluate other factors that may come into play. For instance, it would be nice to know if the chronic neck/back pain following a motor vehicle accident is different from the chronic neck/back pain from work-related injury, versus chronic neck/back pain from osteoarthritis of the spine, a condition associated with overuse and aging. It would also be significant to know what percentage have neck/back pain involving *only* the spine, called *axial pain*, versus the percentage of patients with neck/back pain that radiates to an extremity, called *radicular pain*, or, in the vernacular, sciatica, when referring to pain radiating to the lower extremity. These are key distinctions to make, and the inciting incident, if any, as well as gender, age, race, and ethnicity are also useful to know. Better understanding of epidemiology is the key not only to more effective classification and treatment of pain but also for other issues such as accident prevention on the road and in the workplace, and for ergonomic design.

Epidemiological study is the starting point for the massive work that needs to be done to tease apart the pieces of chronic pain. Once we understand what is happening from the vantage point of populations, we must move on to understanding what is the mechanism of pain in each individual patient. This is a fertile area for research activity, but much of the data that we have is contradictory and confusing. Some of our confusion is due to our poor understanding of the mind-body connection. It is well known that chronic pain triggers the activation of centers of the brain having to do with memory and emotion. Chronic pain in humans is not just a physical and physiological process but also a cognitive, emotional, and spiritual process.

Research has shown that approximately 40 percent of us are going about our daily activities with no pain and a bulging or herniated disc.[7] This was not known over thirty years ago but became apparent with the

---

7   NEJM 331, no. 2 (July 14, 1994): 69–73.

use of MRI and CT scans to help diagnose neck and low back pain. This information was available even earlier, but it was ignored because it didn't mesh well with the understanding at the time.

I used to search the older pain management literature when I was a pain management fellow in training. One day I came across a paper from 1968 that was simply amazing! In the period prior to CT scans, the only diagnostic test for detecting brain lesions was a test called the myelogram. Basically this was an x-ray of a thick dye that was placed in the fluid around the lower spine, called cerebrospinal fluid, which would outline or contrast the spinal fluid from surrounding areas. Since the dye was placed in the lower spine, patients with suspected brain lesions were turned upside down so that their heads were the most dependent or lowest part of the body, thus using gravity to coax the contrast dye into the fluid-filled spaces of the brain. If there was an abnormality in the area of the dye, the possibility of a brain lesion was considered and exploratory neurosurgery planned. Aren't you glad that we have come a long way from that!

At any rate, in the process of performing the myelogram for complaints *related only to the brain,* radiologists noted that in 37 percent of cases there was a herniated lumbar (low back) disc that was not causing pain.[8] This paper was revolutionary, but no one seemed to notice or to care. Surgeons continued to perform discectomies, and sometime spinal fusions with abysmal results. The key point is this: *not every herniated disc is responsible for pain.*

The myelogram, CT scan and MRI are all tests of structure but not of function; therefore, they will only inform of the integrity of structural components but not whether they are responsible for producing pain. This essential point is lost on physicians and patients alike, and you might ignore this rule at your own peril, when out of desperation from the intense suffering from pain you elect to have surgery to correct the herniated disc. The fact that not every herniated disc is responsible for pain is the crux of the decision-making process.

---

8   W. E. Hitselberger and R. M. Written, "Abnormal Myelograms in Asymptomatic Patients," J. Neurosurgery 28 (1968): 204–206.

If not *every* herniated disc causes pain, then which type of herniated disc does cause pain?

The question actually needs to be reframed, and I will return to that briefly. In the middle of my career, I found myself searching for reasons that a herniated disc causes pain, because everyone was convinced that herniated discs are responsible for most cases of low back pain. What is the evidence that herniated discs are responsible for chronic neck and low back pain, and how can we reconcile that evidence with the fact that herniated discs are not the source of pain in every instance?

There are compelling reasons to believe that herniated discs generate pain. Anatomically, they are in close proximity to the nerve roots (figure 3) so that when a disc breaches its normal confines, there is *the potential* for that disc to compress a nerve root, thus inflaming and compressing that nerve root and causing radicular pain. In this case, the disc would have to be demonstrated to show actual nerve compression on MRI. This is not true in many cases of low back pain. The disc can be slightly bulging, without contacting the nerve root, and yet neck/low back pain can still be quite severe. How can this occur?

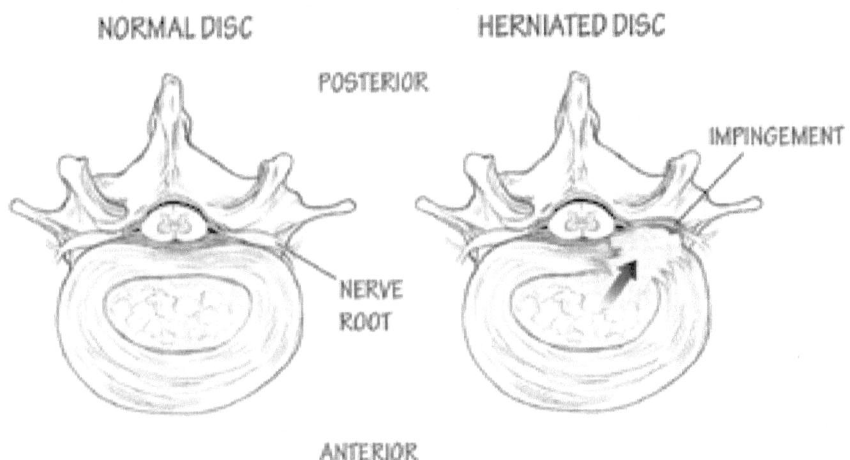

Figure 3. Cross section of normal and herniated disc (arrow is pointing to breach of inner disc and compression of nerve root).

In cases of chronic back pain, sometimes the *only abnormality* on the MRI is a herniated or bulging disc. It is only natural to assume that the cause of the pain is the abnormality on the MRI scan. There are two problems with this reasoning. First, there is not a strong correlation between MRI changes and the experience of pain. In other words, you cannot say that just because there is an abnormal test result, that is the certain cause of pain. Structural abnormality does not imply causation. This is a pervasive problem in medicine, relying on test results to give a complete picture. There are a great number of unnecessary operations and procedures performed on the basis of diagnostic tests. The most reliable way to form a diagnostic impression is to perform the old-fashioned history and physical. I often say that my hands are my most sensitive tools. The remaining tests should be used to help the clinician either support or reject the initial impression. Doctors must make all the pieces of information fit together harmoniously, and without bias, in order for patients to become healthy. Physicians are responsible for being realistic about which therapies have the greatest chance of success.

There is an even more vexing problem with the MRI scan for chronic back pain. What approach am I to take with the patient who has chronic back pain and a normal MRI? Talk about diagnostic dilemmas. Is this patient legitimate in terms of his or her complaints, or is he or she just seeking pain medications? If the MRI is the only factor that determines whether or not the doctor will believe that you have pain, you will have great difficulty convincing him or her that you are in pain with a *normal* MRI, assuming other causes have been ruled out. We have seen some dishonest patients who seek entrée to pain management services by providing false MRIs. What should be particularly irksome to anyone who considers this is that we (medicine and society) have created a situation that a positive MRI is the arbiter of who is a genuine person in pain. Nothing could be farther from the truth. My goal is to demonstrate that chronic pain can exist in the presence or absence of the objective radiological testing available today.

Another reason that the discs are considered to be a source of pain is the unique features of disc material. Discs are meant to be the functional shock absorbers of the spine. They are also spacers between the bones of the vertebrae that allow the nerve roots to travel out to the body unimpeded, without compression (figure 4).

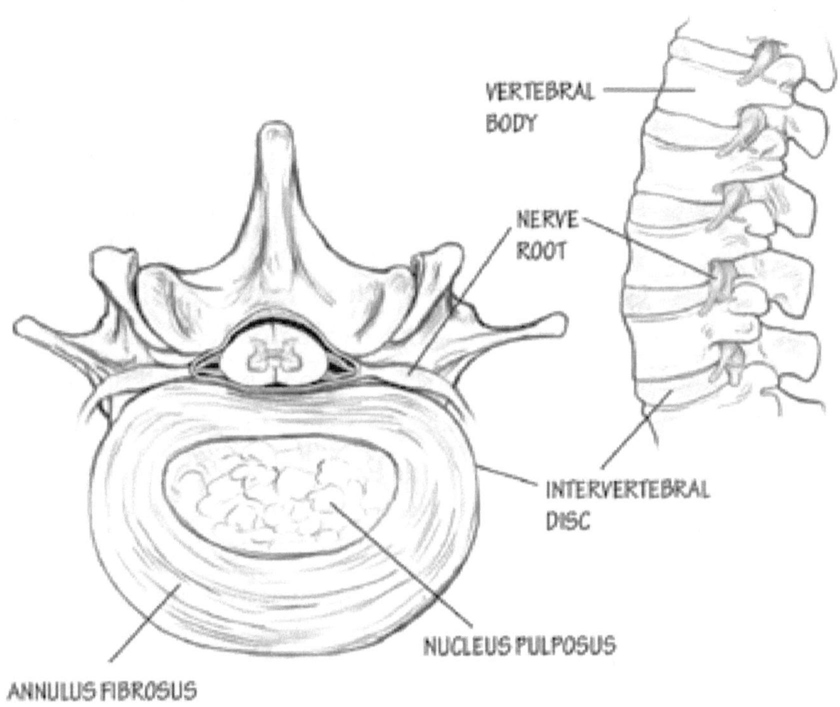

Figure 4. Cross section and side views of relationship of disc to the spine and nerve roots (notice in the lateral or side view that the disc provides both cushioning between the vertebral bodies as well as height in order to allow nerve roots to freely exit the spinal canal without impingement).

Structurally, discs are like those candies, Mentos, that have a hard outside and a soft gelatinous inside. The outer hard shell of the intervertebral disc is known as the *annulus fibrosis* and the soft inner portion is the *nucleus pulposus* (figure 4). If the outer annulus is breached, the inner material leaks out. This is the condition some refer to as a torn annulus. The disc itself has no blood supply, and the nucleus pulposus consists of glycoproteins, a relatively inert material. From early development of the body, this inner disc material is isolated from the rest of the body and therefore has the potential to be recognized by the immune system as a foreign protein, thus allowing an inflammatory response to be set up, should that protein come in contact with the environment outside the disc. There are good research studies to support this theory. The nerve roots are very close to the discs. If the disc is disrupted and some disc fluid is spilled on a nerve root, there is the possibility for an inflammatory response to be set up in the area of the nerve root, causing pain throughout the distribution of that nerve root, defined as *radiculitis*. Of all the reasons to consider the disc as a source of pain, the concepts of leaking disc and nerve root compression by herniated discs are most plausible. However, while a leaking disc can be demonstrated radiologically via a test called *discography*, the next step of demonstrating or imaging inflamed nerve tissue in live subjects has never been achieved. Hopefully in the future, the imaging of inflamed or damaged nerves will become a reality, thus giving us an important tool for diagnosis and treatment of all types of chronic pain.

A problem with the leaky disc theory is that most of chronic neck/back pain is axial and not radicular, meaning the most common types of chronic neck/LBP (low back pain) are restricted to the spine; it is much less common for a nerve root to cause pain throughout an extremity, and even when an extremity is painful, the possibility of pseudo-radiculopathy, pain that seems to be radicular, but in actuality is not, must be entertained (Chapter 6).

There is another silent epidemic that causes back pain with no involvement of the discs. The silent epidemic of osteoarthritis along with other rheumatologic diseases affecting the spine will be discussed in Chapter 8.

* * * * *

In the field of epidemiology, we speak of false positives and false negatives. A false positive is a test that shows a misleading positive finding that the clinician may feel compelled to act upon. The case of patients presenting false MRIs is a good example, but so is the fact that 40 percent of people without chronic low back pain have herniated discs on the MRI. We can never tell just by looking at the MRI alone whether a given disc is causing pain.

A false negative is the case of a patient with chronic low back pain (LBP) who is told that there is no reason for his or her complaints due to a negative or normal MRI report of the spine. I am particularly concerned about these patients, because often they are branded as phonies, drug seekers, or malingerers. Some are, but many are not.

How many times in life are things not what they seem? How many people are sitting in prison for crimes they did not commit? If not for innovation in DNA analysis, many of these people would remain unjustly incarcerated. What about our politicians who promise to represent us with transparency and selflessness? In some cases, this is true, but often we feel cheated and are disappointed. Societal norms can fluctuate like a pendulum, but a person's individual experience tends not to fluctuate so much. None of us are able to experience the inner world of another person, and ultimately the best we can ever do is to accumulate enough data in an objective fashion in order to come as close to the truth as humanly possible. Nowhere are these points more relevant than the ways in which we interface and interact with chronic pain patients.

Chronic pain as a condition can be a personal, societal, and medical nightmare. Anyone caught up in this whirlwind who is truly suffering and not manipulating the system is deserving of our sympathy and compassion.

In this chapter, you have learned the following:

- The difficulties and challenges involved in medical decision making
- In medicine, as in life, things are not always as they appear
- That not every abnormality of the soft tissue of the spine seen on MRI is clinically significant
- Basic concepts of epidemiology
- Hypotheses regarding the mechanisms of back pain caused by disc herniation

Chapter 3

The Architecture of the Spine

The Vertebrae and Spinal Joints in Sickness and in Health

When I began my practice, I wondered why patients would seek chiropractic care before consulting with a pain physician. It seemed to me that the manipulation of spinal joints had nothing to do with treating herniated discs, which were felt to be the likely cause of chronic back pain. As for the patients who sought chiropractic care, I assumed that they just didn't like the idea of having injections to treat back pain, unless they were desperate, and for that I could not blame them.

I also recall having a long debate with the director of my pain-management training program over whether pain causes psychological issues or vice versa. This is a fertile area for discussion, and a good clinician tries to keep in mind the psychological state of the patient under all circumstances. Studies find that in many cases of chronic pain, depression *results from* the loss of abilities and relationships associated with chronic pain.[9], [10]

---

9   "The Temporal Relation between Pain and Depression: Results from the Longitudinal Aging Study, Amsterdam," Psychosomatic Med 74, no. 9 (Nov–Dec 2012): 948–951.

10   "Clinical Rounds," OB-Gyn News (May 15, 2005): 34.

I think it is unlikely for a person who is independent one day and then has a serious injury and is subsequently chronically in pain to desire to be dependent on others and magnify or fabricate symptoms, although I am sure it does happen, especially when litigation and money are involved. There is, however, great value to psychological interventions in pain management in terms of teaching patients coping strategies for dealing with pain as well as therapeutic intervention for situations such as traumatic brain injury and post-traumatic stress disorder. Of course, doctors must always remember that patients come with all of their existing psychological conditions. They may have underlying personality disorders, potential for addiction, and neuroses that can become amplified by any illness, particularly chronic pain, due to the fact that pain is a very subjective experience with little in the way of objective evidence. For this reason alone, I feel that there is tremendous value in the input of psychological therapists in the treatment of chronic pain.

Over my years of practice, I have questioned the value of other therapies. It is not enough for a treatment to be effective; I also want to understand *why* it is effective. If I can understand the mechanism of why a treatment works, I can transfer that information from one patient to another. In medicine, our understanding of illness and disease is always changing. In order to maintain competency in my field, over the years I have taken several cadaver courses, in which doctors can learn while avoiding causing pain or discomfort, with the objective of learning new procedures to help relieve chronic pain. I had performed several thousand epidural steroid injections in my career to treat the pain coming from the injured discs, but I had to agree with one of my internal medicine colleagues who once said to me, "I don't mind referring patients to you, but in many cases they just don't seem to get better." Ouch! I was not much more effective than the other health care professionals I was critical of.

At one memorable course, I refreshed performance of some procedures I had learned during my training, but one of the instructors from the Southwest casually mentioned that he had tremendous results treating the posterior (rear) joints of the spine in cases of chronic neck and back pain known as the *facet joints*. I listened intently but rolled my eyes, thinking that this doctor was just misguided. If the disc is herniated, how could the facet joints, which are anatomically not close to the herniated disc, be responsible for chronic pain? In anatomical terms, this did not make sense, since it had always seemed to most pain specialists that herniated discs are the most likely culprit for low back pain. It took me many more years to figure out that he had found a valid, effective approach to chronic pain. Once I considered the posterior facet joints to be a significant cause of pain, I had to reassess the value of other treatments of back pain, such as surgery.

Did you know that where you live can determine the type of treatment you will receive? In an article in the *Washington Post* several years ago, there was an article entitled "When Geography Influences Treatment Options."[11] Low back pain is treated surgically more frequently on the West coast of Florida, while on the East coast of Florida low back pain is treated more conservatively and with less surgery. This is true in many other areas of the country as well (graph 1).

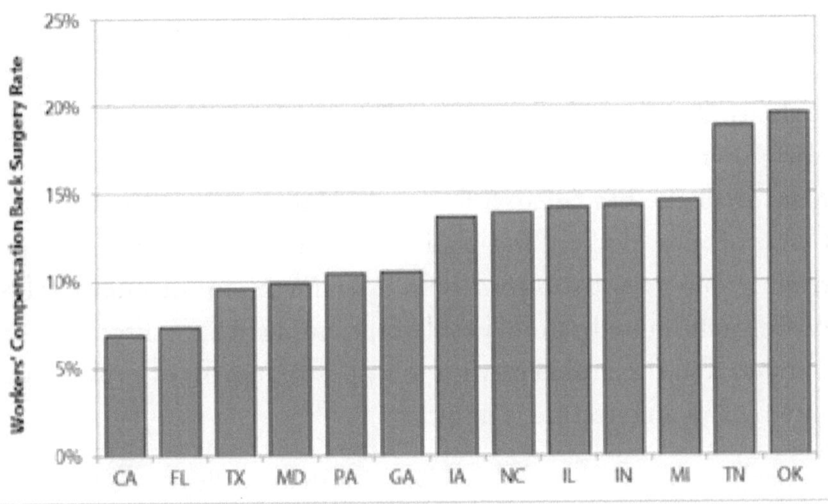

Graph 1.Incidence of back surgery by state for workers' compensation claimants (with permission of WCRI).

---

11   Washington Post (July 25, 2005).

There are many reasons for this disparity, but suffice it to say chronic pain patients are easily convinced to have back surgery. In fact, due to their suffering and disability, in many cases it is difficult to convince chronic neck and low back pain patients *not* to have surgery. There is an air of desperation that pervades many of these doctor-patient interactions, so it is not surprising that the result can be surgery that is not necessarily warranted. There are, of course, certain specific instances when surgery is necessary, which I will discuss in Chapter 9, but in general, it is not advisable to operate for chronic pain in the absence of any other neurological symptoms.

When I think about the way that chronic pain sufferers prefer to seek treatment, the acronym HANDS is a useful mnemonic. Since most patients in pain start out with the chiropractor, the H stands for *hands*, for either massage or manipulation of the joints. Next the patient will move on to A for activity exercises and stretching, usually supervised, in physical therapy. In many cases this will be helpful, but if not, they will progress to N for *needles*, either acupuncture or interventional pain management, then D for denervation or neuroaugmentation, which alter the ability of nerves to transmit pain. This includes RFA or radiofrequency ablation, and spinal cord stimulation, discussed in Chapter 11. And finally, if all else has failed, S for *surgical* intervention. From the point of view of most doctors and patients, this is a logical progression. We certainly don't want someone with a strained joint or pulled muscle, relatively self-limited painful problems, running to have surgery. In order to understand the problems with this approach, a bit of explanation of anatomy and architecture is in order.

When I was a preteenager, I had two toys that I really enjoyed. Being the oldest male with three younger sisters, I spent much of my time occupied with my Legos and also the Visible Man, which was a kind of anatomical model encased in plastic, within which I could take apart and put together various organ systems. My favorite part was the skeletal system. It just seemed so creepy and elegant at the same time, just perfect for a young man of ten or eleven. The Legos caused me to reflect on design and the most efficient use of space, and I think if I hadn't gone to medical school, architecture or mathematical modeling would have been my profession.

In college, I majored in biology, and we spent a great deal of time learning about the formation and architecture of the body from its earliest stages. We were taught that "ontogeny recapitulates phylogeny", meaning that our form, which comes about through the complex genetic, molecular biologic, and cellular interactions of embryology, is a throwback to the evolutionary process. For example, the bones of the forearm are related to the bone structure in the wing of a bird. Since my time in college, this theory has been largely discredited due to the fact that these tissues derive from different tissue lines and are not biologically related. I think that is good news because whether there is a Creator or there are evolutionary forces at play, consider that there are only a finite number of efficient, functional designs for the different parts of the body. In actuality, the choices for performance of a particular function such as locomotion or grasping are quite limited. My professors deserve credit though, because they implanted in my mind forever that structure (or form) and function in biological systems must go together. This was my guide to a better understanding of neck/back mechanics and causes of chronic pain.

In life, in order to understand the "what" of something, one first needs to understand the "how" and the "why". I don't know if this is true for other disciplines, but it is certainly true for all meaningful scientific inquiry. Why are we constructed the way that we are? Does it confer some advantage relative to the lower mammals? Does our architecture pose unique problems relative to other animals? On the basis of our structure, are there activities to be avoided, and are there measures to be taken to prevent damage? What then is the description of the mechanism of chronic neck and low back pain? These essential questions are at the nexus of modern anthropology, biomechanics, and biology.

Most of the salient differences between man and animal, in terms of skeletal structure, are due to the fact that we are the only full-time two-legged animals. We don't use our hands at all to help us walk, and our poor feet are meant to bear the brunt of the mass that balances above them. The arches of the feet are meant to be shock absorbers for the spine, just as the discs are, so if your arches are fallen, sometimes the only intervention required for treatment of chronic back pain is to use orthotics in the shoes. Solutions can sometimes be that simple.

Our bodies require a support system to allow for upright posture as well as the fluctuations inherent in movement, such as walking and bending, while at the same time supporting legs, arms, and the head. Add to this the bellows system needed for the lungs and the protection from damage that the internal organs and brain require (rib cage, cranium), and one can appreciate the complexity of design of the human skeleton. As part of that design, we also require a system for electrical transmission, plumbing, heating, and cooling.

The electrical system of the body is known as the *nervous system*. It is not simply a bunch of wires that run throughout the body. It is rather a *biological system* that interacts with other systems in the body, with the spine as a relay station, and the brain as the master integrator and controller. The main way that nerves differ from wires is that if you damage or cut a nerve, one end continues to be attached and responsive to the central system. This type of issue is dealt with frequently in the field of pain management.

Once the skeletal system is assembled, how is the nervous system integrated? In our development, the brain and spinal cord are formed prior to the bones, joints, and muscles, so actually the motherboard, microchips, and sensors are all in place initially and later protected within cartilage and bone. For our purposes, it is convenient to think of the nerves of the spine as encased within the vertebral bodies that make up the spinal cord. The nerve roots emanate from the spinal cord to provide sensory input and motor (locomotive) output to the rest of the body (figure 5).

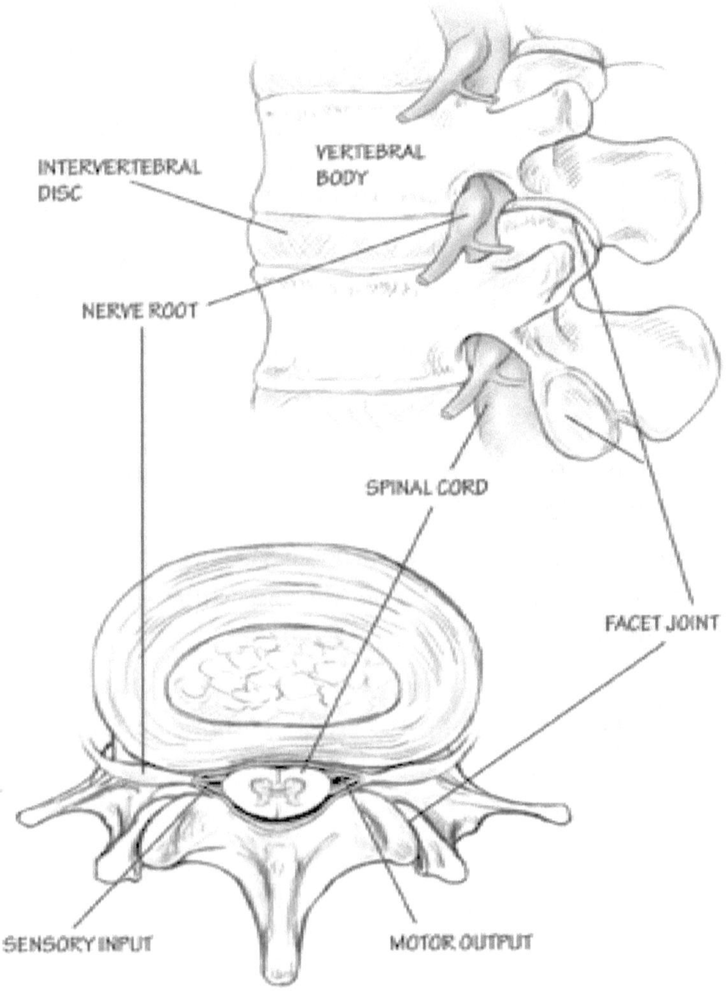

Figure 5. Relationships of intervertebral discs, spine, nerve roots, and facet joints in cross section and lateral views.

Clearly this is an oversimplification, but like any good representation, it helps explain a great deal. It is logical to ask, why is it necessary for the spine and brain to be encased in bone? There is a class of creatures called *invertebrates* that have nervous systems but no spines. They can only creep and crawl along very slowly. Our nervous systems are vastly advanced and developed in terms of the ability to constantly monitor the environment and respond to it, so that the central nervous structures, better known as the *central nervous system* (CNS), needed to be encased in bone for protection. If our spines were not protected in this fashion, we would constantly be subjected to serious injury, resulting in muscle weakness or paralysis, and a constant barrage of sensory insults. An extra measure of cushioning is afforded to our central nervous system by a fluid-filled sac around the sensitive nerve structures of the brain and spine. The fluid is known as *cerebrospinal fluid*, and the sac is called the *meninges* (figure 6). A fluid barrier is a very effective way to cushion the effects of outer forces. Outside the central nervous system, consisting of the spine and brain, the peripheral nerves are not encased in bone or fluid, thus enabling our bodies to have the flexibility to rapidly respond to perceived threats from the environment.

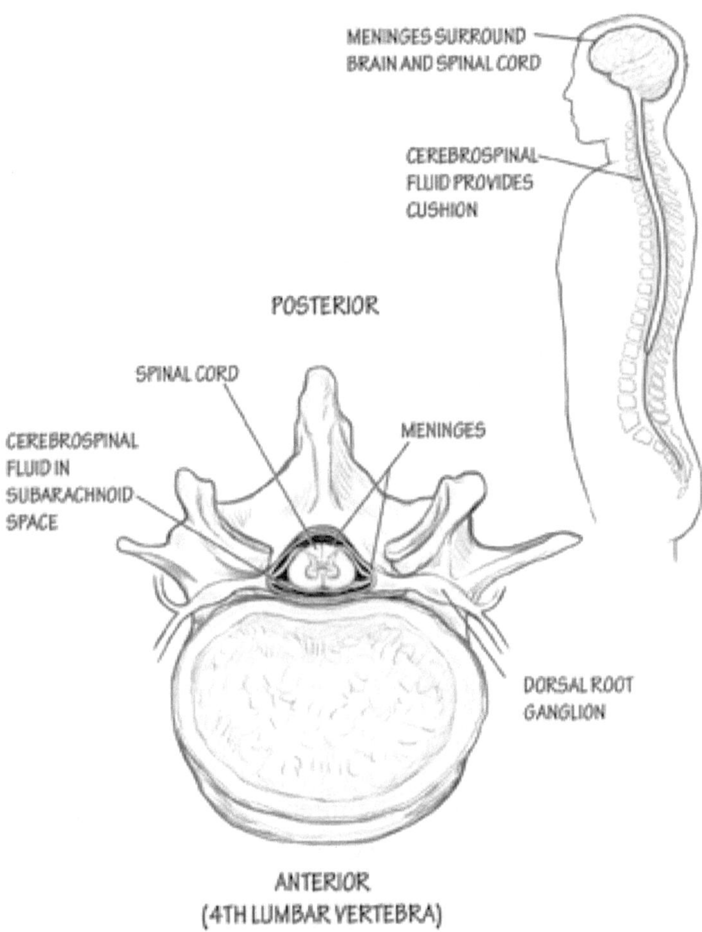

Figure 6. Important structures of the body containing nerve tissue in many cases are encased in fluid and membranes, known as meninges, and bone. This can be considered protective packaging that protects against various outside forces. The fluid functions as a shock absorber, and the bone provides physical protection from sharp objects or blunt trauma.

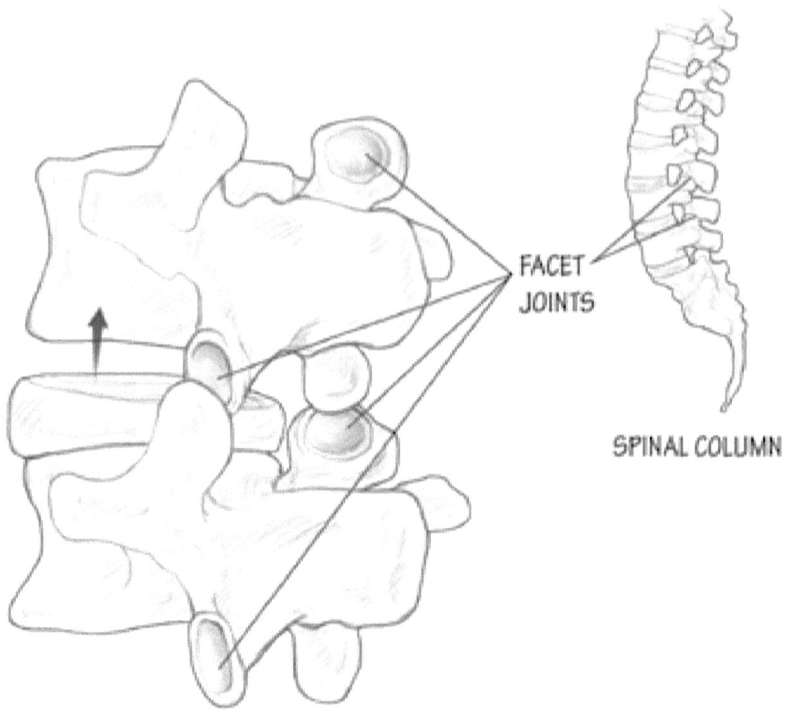

Figure 7. Relationship between the intervertebral discs and facet joints (each vertebral body rests like a tripod on one broad anterior intervertebral disc and two posterior facet joints).

While on the topic of flexibility, let's focus again on the architecture of the body. If our bones were fused to each other, we would be quite stiff and unable to bend, torque, or rotate our bones relative to each other, thus limiting mobility. Without the hinging effect that is afforded by the joints, it would be impossible to respond to dangers in the environment that require a fight-or-flight response, and our species would have died out long ago. Our joints are so important that our existence hinges on them. There are several types of joints throughout the body, allowing for a range of motion specific to each joint. In the case of the spine, each vertebral body sits on top of three joints. There is the large joint in the front known as the *intervertebral disc*, which we have discussed, but there are also two joints to the rear of the vertebral body, which are known as *facet joints* (figure 7). The vertebrae of your body essentially stack one upon the other, much like building blocks or stacking chairs. This arrangement allows for your spine to bend forward, backward, to the sides, and also to rotate, most effectively in the cervical or neck area. It is interesting to note that each of the vertebrae have different shapes that allow for some unique features (figure 8). The intervertebral discs also add height to the spinal column, allowing for the unimpeded travel of the nerve roots to the periphery (figure 4). The discs also act as shock absorbers for the central or axial portion of the skeletal system. This fact is of importance in the discussion of high-velocity trauma.

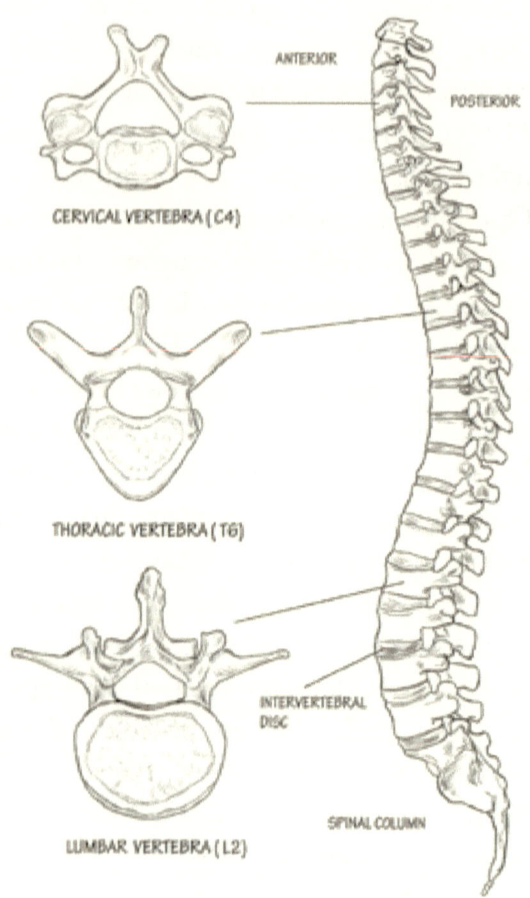

Figure 8. While each vertebral body rests on one intervertebral disc and two facet joints, the shape of the vertebrae differ in the cervical,- thoracic and lumbar spines. Cervical vertebrae are smaller and lack transverse processes. The carotid artery traverses the cervical vertebrae—notice the two foramina, or holes, in the anterior cervical vertebrae. Thoracic vertebrae articulate with the ribs segmentally, and the force from damage to the ribs can be transmitted back to thoracic facet joints. Lumbar vertebrae are the widest and broadest vertebrae and bear much of the forces that act on the spine.

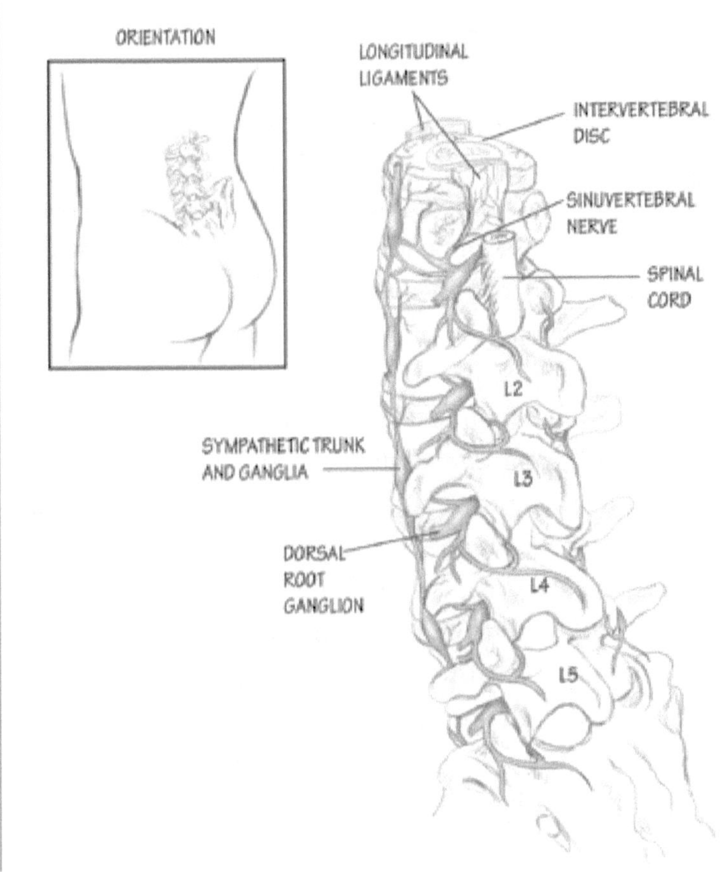

Figure 9. Relationship between autonomic and somatic nervous systems. The sympathetic chain runs lateral and anterior to the vertebral bodies and controls involuntary functions for the internal organs in close proximity; the somatic nervous system is contained within the bony confines of the spinal canal and emerges at each spinal level to form the nerve roots.

Looking at an anatomical specimen we cannot always determine its exact purpose and function. We need to examine and measure the structure under live conditions in order to know the exact role of that tissue in the body. Since nerves can be either *afferent* (sensory) or *efferent* (motor or other response to stimulus) and also either *somatic* (supplying the skeletal muscles, bones, and joints) or autonomic (supplying and regulating the internal organs, smooth muscle found in heart, lungs, and blood vessels, temperature regulation, neuroendocrine function, vibration, and position senses), it is difficult to identify the type and role of a nerve just by looking at it. Somatic nerves are the source of our ability to move and to sense pain from the external environment. These fibers are known as a *delta fibers*, and transmit pain rapidly with a sharp quality. Autonomic nerves, by contrast, allow for the unconscious fine-tuning of the body. *Autonomic nerves* control temperature regulation to and from the environment, as well as the release of hormones and digestive juices and sense pain from the internal organs and the internal environment. These sensory fibers are known as *c fibers* and transmit pain slowly, spasmodically, and can have a burning or lancinating quality. They autonomic nervous system also influences heart rate and cardiac output, blood flow and respiration, and most important for our discussion, vibration and the ability for the brain to nonconsciously sense the position of joints in order to maintain balance.

There is a major difference between the intervertebral disc and the two facet joints. The intervertebral disc does not have any significant somatic nerve innervation, while the facet joints are richly innervated by the first branch of the (somatic) spinal nerve root, a branch of which is called the *medial branch*, which runs posteriorly and provides innervation to both the facet joints and the paraspinous muscles. The *sinuvertebral nerve*, which is *autonomic* in its derivation, innervates the outer layers of the disc and vertebrae circumferentially (figures 9, 10, 11). Our spine has a mechanism for sensing and maintaining our sense of balance and, with the subconscious, awareness of our center of gravity. [12]

---

12   For more complete discussion of this topic see, Propriception: The Forgotten Sixth Sense, Spine and Proprioception, M. G. Karakaya, and I. C. Karakaya, OMICS eBook Group. www.esciencecentral.org/ebooks.

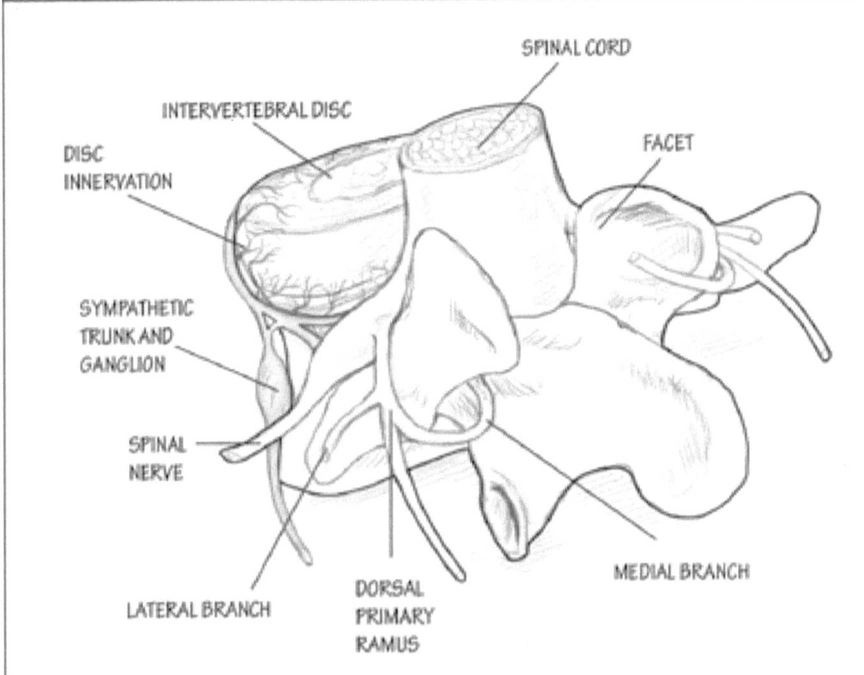

Figure 10. Individual spinal segment showing relationships of the innervation of the intervertebral disc and that of the facet joints in the lumbar region. As demonstrated, the facet joint is innervated by the first posterior branch of the nerve root, known as the dorsal ramus. This is significant because the implication is that the facets joints have somatic innervation similar to joints, muscles, tendons, and bones. Thus pain from facet joint injury will have a dull, aching quality with occasional sharp component, similar to injury to bone, muscle, tendon, or joint in the periphery. It is also significant to note that the majority of intervertebral disc innervation seen in the diagram emanates from the sympathetic chain. This may indicate that the role of the disc innervation may not be to detect or sense pain, but rather to assess and report the position of the spine relative to its orientation to the rest of the body and the environment.

We are richly innervated in the area around our discs and vertebrae by the *multiple sensors* that send information to the brain that informs it of our location and position in space. This is also true of our extremities and is particularly important for maintaining proper skeletal balance and posture.

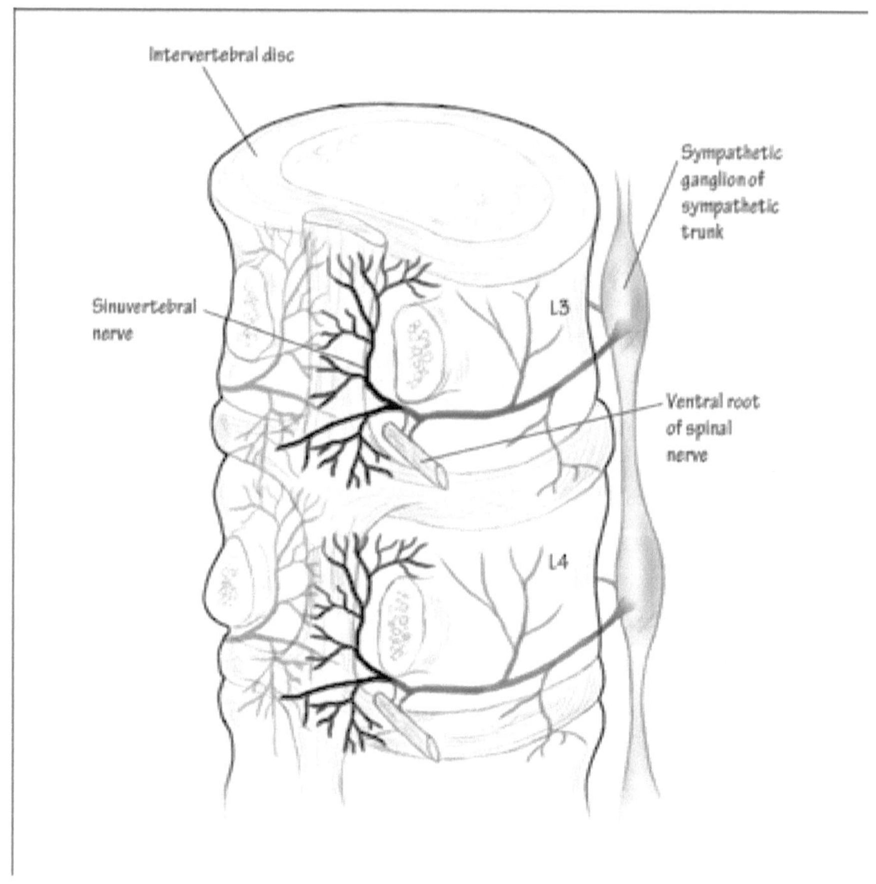

Figure 11. The sinuvertebral nerve, which is a branch of the autonomic nervous system, sends many branches from the sympathetic chain to the periphery of the spine with multiple arborizations to the outer surface of the discs, bone, and ligaments of the spine. This extensive innervation

may be an indication of the potential for this system to sense the position of the spine itself. Injury to this system would produce diffuse pain that can be burning or lancinating in nature, not at all similar to the somatic pain experienced with injury to the facet joints. The presence and diffuse arrangement of multiple sensory points lends validity to the theory that the sympathetic chain has a positional sensing function for the spine.

The *sinuvertebral nerve*, which innervates the disc and vertebrae, is derived from autonomic branches. Since the sharp component of pain that radiates down extremities (radicular pain) is associated with the somatic nervous system, we can be fairly certain that structures innervated by the sinuvertebral nerve will not generate the same kind of pain that one would have in the extremities but rather a burning, spasmodic, diffused aching type of pain associated with irritation or blockage of the internal organs if, indeed, any pain is generated. In fact, it is not clear as to whether nerves to injured discs sense pain; remember that 40% of the population has evidence of disc herniation and presumably disruption of the associated nerves close to the disc without any pain. Patients are usually able to do a good job of localizing the fairly constant dull, aching somatic pain that can have a sharp component radiating into an extremity, but it is more difficult to describe and localize pain that derives from internal organs.

It is not a stretch to consider that the spine would be innervated on its outside with sensors just like any other internal organ. What then would be the purpose of autonomic innervation from the sinuvertebral nerve to the spine? Perhaps the simplest understanding of the anatomy and function of the autonomic nerves associated with innervation of the outer portion of the spine would be to provide position sense or proprioception, and not the sensation of pain from a herniated disc.[13] In order for us to maintain our upright position through walking, running, or even performing household chores, it is logical to make the assumption that just as our muscles have sensors of position that are relayed to the spine and then the brain, so

---

13 An indirect proof of this is that vascular disruption of the posterior spinal cord (where the sinuvertebral nerve is located), will cause balance problems but anterior spinal vascular syndromes do not affect balance.

too the axial spine, which can be thought of as a "stick" that our cranium and limbs are attached to and in a sense suspended by and from, would require sensors to transmit a sense of position from around the spine for determination of center of gravity and moment. Only by sensing the center of gravity can the brain provide feedback to muscles, providing the resulting balance for maintaining upright posture that is stable (figure 12). In my opinion, *a possible function of the nerves that are found on the surface of the vertebrae and disc is maintenance of balance and position and not the sensation of pain.*

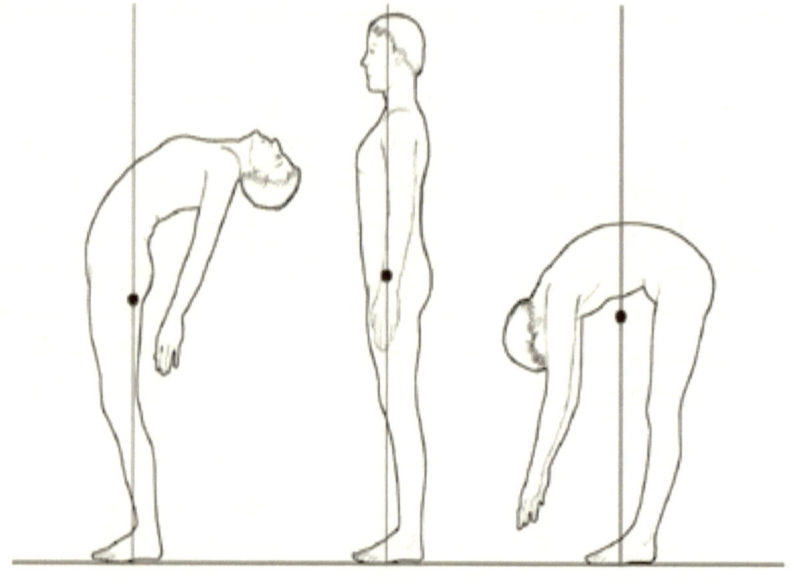

Figure 12. Center of gravity, position sense and the spine. This is a complex system involving the inner ear, eyes, and visual and balance centers of the brain. The autonomic system represented by the sinuvertebral nerve represents the sensory part of this system, which sends impulses to specialized sections of the brain. In this sense, the autonomic innervation of the spine resembles the autonomic innervation of the (other) internal organs.

Unfortunately, many clinicians and researchers have concluded that the presence of the sinuvertebral nerve is evidence that the disc can "feel pain." This assumption is likely unfounded since, as I have stated, 40 percent of us have an asymptomatic bulging or herniated disc that we are unable to detect throughout our daily activities. It is reasonable to assume that just as these discs are disrupted and not painful, so too may the nerves that innervate them become disrupted and not painful. Logic and consistency would dictate that the nerves innervating the disc are not generally responsible for the sensation of pain but rather the sensation of a totally different type—position and balance.

In order for chronic pain to exist, there must be a sensory nerve that is damaged, irritated or inflamed. This is true for both the somatic and autonomic sensory systems. (An example of an autonomic sensory abnormality is diabetic neuropathy.) The absence of a somatic sensory nerve that innervates the intervertebral discs indicates that there is no somatic sensory apparatus for detecting damage that has occurred to an intervertebral disc. Any pain sensed at the area of the disc should be similar to pain emanating from internal organs, and we know that this is not what our patients are experiencing.

One could argue that the nerve root that emanates from the spinal cord can sense damage to the intervertebral disc. This would be true only if a disc was sitting upon a nerve root, or if the disc material could somehow reach the nerve root and cause inflammation. As I have mentioned, the outer part of the disc can become disrupted, and the inner nucleus pulposus material can spill on to the nerve root, causing inflammation in the area of the nerve root and possibly producing pain.

While this may be a plausible explanation for chronic back pain, one can ask why there is not consistently additional pain following disc surgery when the disc has been surgically disrupted, and potentially an inflammatory response set up by the remaining disc material. In recent years, percutaneous (through the skin) discectomy has become a popular way of removing disc material.

It involves removing a small piece of disc via needle, thereby relieving pressure in the disc. Why is there not additional pain caused by this procedure? By the very nature of placing a needle in the center of a disc, the disc is disrupted, leading to additional leaking of disc material. It seems that disc material may not be as irritating to nerve roots as originally thought. In fact, in recent years it has been shown that herniated discs exhibit characteristics of hysteresis, meaning that small increases of volumes within the disc which we refer to as a herniated disc, causes much greater than expected increases in pressure by the disc on the nerve roots, thus supporting theories of pain which is caused by mechanical pressure from herniated disc material. Sometimes in science a hypothesis seems sound, but when tested in the real world, things do not add up. The best hypotheses account for all possibilities under all conditions.

In this chapter, you have learned the following:

- Why we are constructed in the fashion that we are, and the influence of upright posture on our architecture

- The ways in which the body protects sensitive structures such as the spine, brain, and developing fetus from injury, such as the spine, brain, and developing fetus

- The importance of our joints in allowing us to respond rapidly to threats in our environment, and why much chronic pain involves the joints

- The two complementary nervous systems that run through your body

- The importance of feedback from the spine to the brain of position sense (of the spine) and the possible role of the sinuvertebral nerve in this function

Chapter 4

Facet Joint Arthritis versus Facet Syndrome

Is It Real or Virtual?

There is one last candidate in the search for causes of mechanical chronic neck and low back pain. The facet joints described previously are particularly sensitive to damage and injury from a variety of causes ranging from arthritis to trauma. Why are these joints so vulnerable? The facet joints, like most joints in the body, are susceptible to damage from overuse, excessive weight bearing, and repetitive minor trauma. They are a site where inflammation can accumulate and cause arthritis. As the inflammation increases, there is the potential for compression of the nerve root due to the close proximity of the facet joint and nerve root. The fact that the facet joint has its own somatic nerve supply called the *medial branch* supports the concept that it will be a site more likely responsible for generation of somatic pain than the intervertebral disc, which is not somatically innervated.

In cases of trauma such as flexion-hyperextension injury, also known as *whiplash injury*, the facet joints are very susceptible to damage. In the flexion phase, when the neck or low back is moving forward, the intervertebral disc becomes pinched, thus causing the posterior rupture of the broad-based intervertebral disc, resulting in a bulging or herniated disc (figure 13).

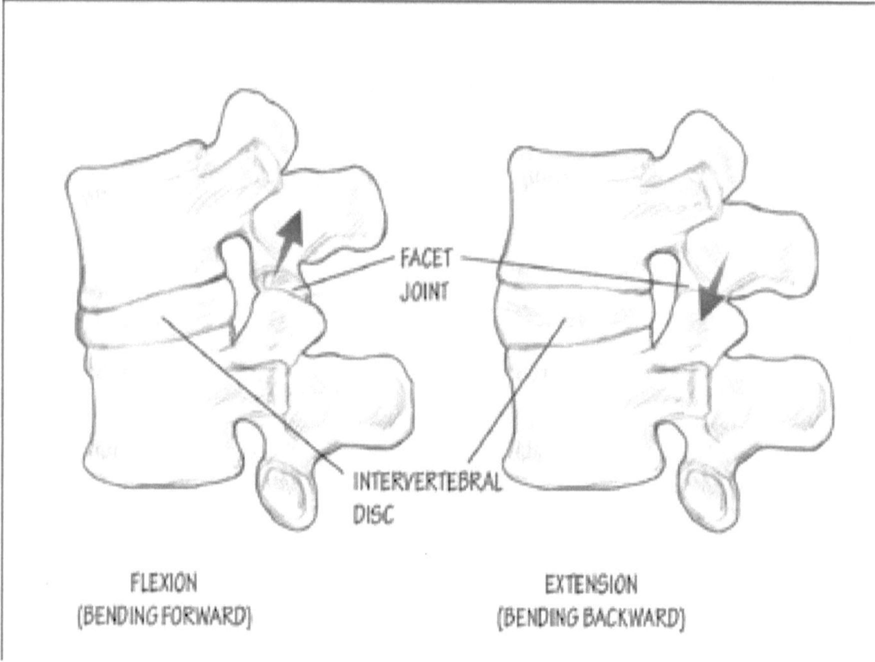

Figure 13. The lumbar facet joints in flexion and extension. Pressure in the facet joints rises dramatically in extension, while pressure in the intervertebral disc rises with flexion.

In the extension phase, a great deal of pressure is placed on the much smaller area facet joints, causing the facet joints and the small nerves supplying them to come under greater force. This force not only can damage the facet joint but can also stretch the fine medial branch nerves that supply the joint. The stretched nerve and/or damaged facet joint begins to send a barrage of painful messages through the spine to the brain. In cases where the joint or medial branch do not heal, from either arthritis or injury, a chronic painful situation is likely. The scenario I have put forth here conforms with the definition of chronic pain, but now there is an anatomical and physiological explanation. This is truly pain that lasts beyond the normal healing phase without any useful purpose.

But there is much more. As I stated, understanding the "why" of what is happening is of critical importance and will give clues as to what is truly happening. In a world in which we have become accustomed to trusting our senses, "seeing is believing." When a process requires the input of our imagination, which possibly contradicts what we see, we are instant critics and skeptics. I think that a good dose of skepticism is essential, *but* I am also willing to suspend disbelief when my preconceived notions do not fit facts in the real world. If it is true that the intervertebral discs are the cause of most chronic low back pain, then their partial removal should resolve chronic pain, and that is not usually the case.

Now imagine a different world where things are *not exactly* the way they seem ...

Case Study 1

A forty-five-year-old white female was the driver of a vehicle that was rear-ended by another vehicle eighteen months ago. She sustained a whiplash injury to her neck and low back in the accident, without loss of consciousness. She was seen in the local emergency room, and x-rays of the neck and low back failed to reveal any fracture. Since the accident, she has difficulty finding a comfortable position to sleep in, and it is also difficult to lift, bend, or sit for prolonged periods. She has had no pain, numbness, or weakness in the extremities. There is back stiffness upon awakening. The pain feels like a constant soreness with pressure in the neck and low back. She describes her pain as moderate to severe, with some relief from Vicodin two to three times a day. Her physical exam is significant only for decreased range of motion in extension in the cervical and lumbar spines, and pain to palpation over the cervical and lumbar facet joints, and positive facet joint loading. Straight leg raising test is negative. MRI of the cervical spine was normal, and MRI of the lumbar spine shows a L4-L5 bulging disc and L5-S1 herniated disc. She has been treated with chiropractic manipulation, massage and physical therapy, and a series of three lumbar and three cervical epidural steroid injections, with only brief periods of relief. She is contemplating low back surgery because she feels that everything she has tried has not worked.

This is a typical patient seen in my office. She is frustrated and upset because before the accident she could keep up with her kids. Now her job performance and relationships are suffering due to sleep deprivation and pain, and now the pain just seems to linger with no end in sight, and she is tired of popping pain pills. She has come to see me as the "specialist of last resort" prior to surgery.

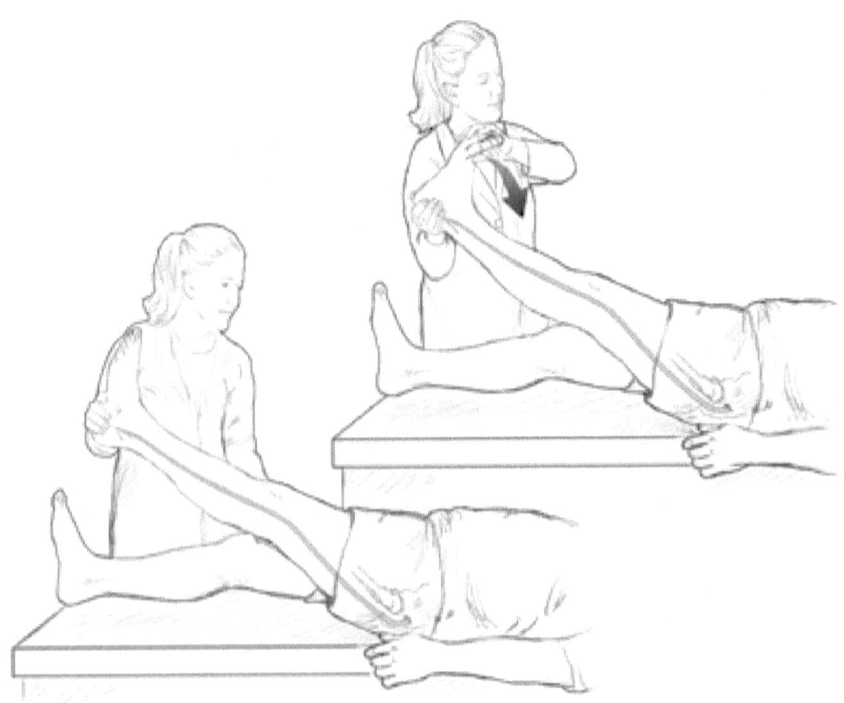

Figure 14. Straight leg raising test (SLR) demonstrates radicular pain only if pain radiates from low back or hip down to the ankle. The raising of the leg places stretching forces on the lower lumbar nerve roots. If the nerve root is irritated, pain will radiate through the entire distribution of the nerve root. If there is only pain in the hamstring muscles or only in the hip, knee, or ankle this is not a positive SLR test, and no evidence of radiculopathy.

It would seem that the bulging and herniated discs are responsible for the back pain. But something doesn't fit. There is no pain in her legs, which would indicate nerve root irritation or compression, and tests that elicit the pain of nerve root irritation, such as straight leg raising (figure 14), were also negative. In addition, the neck pain is of a similar quality to the low back pain but without any herniated discs. She has had multiple epidural injections with no relief. There are two indications that the facet joints are injured. First is the decreased range of motion in extension, a position in which the facet joints undergo pressure, and also there is frank pain with application of pressure at the affected facet joints in the neck and low back. The MRI shows a herniated disc, but it does not appear from my examination that there is any nerve root irritation, which would be expected if pain is from disc disruption.

The facet joints become painful only when there is inflammation of the joint (facet arthropathy, figure 15) or damage to the medial branch nerve that innervates the facet joints (facet syndrome, figure 16), which is true in this case. In both cases, though, the pain will be identical because the sensation of a damaged (medial) nerve is indistinguishable from the pain of an injured (facet) joint.

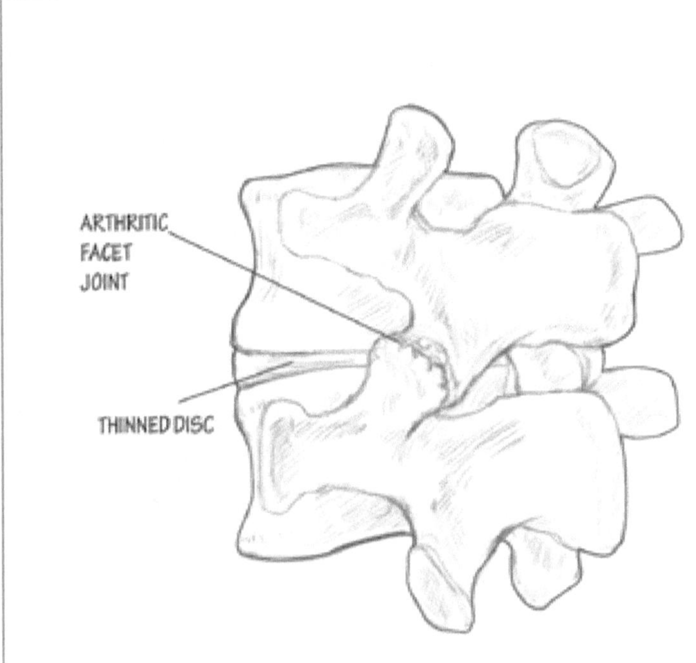

Figure 15. Evidence of damage or injury to facet joint, resulting in arthritis and inflammation of the facet joint.

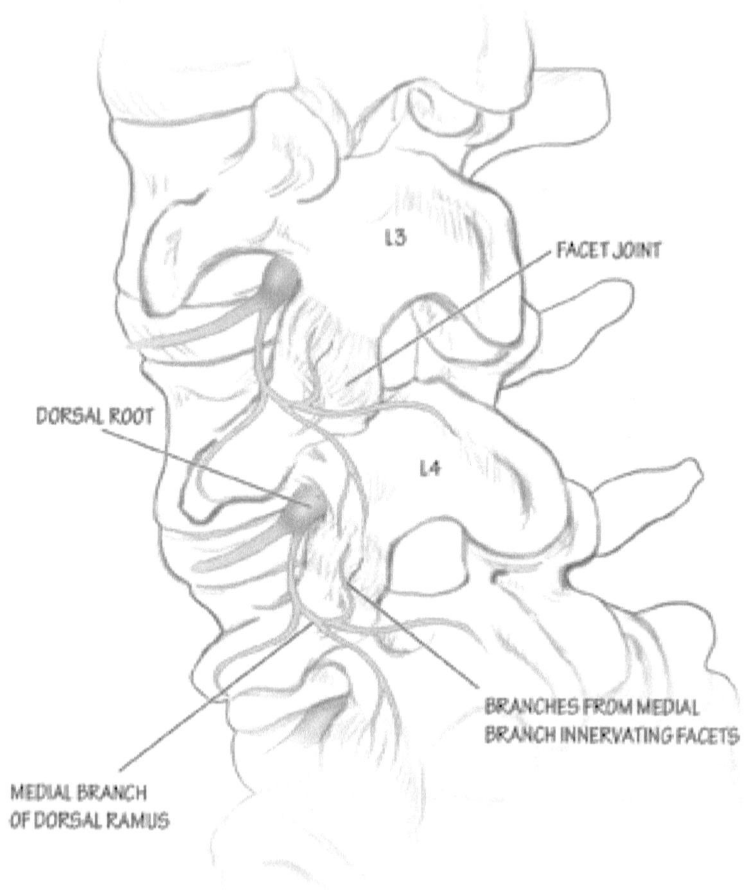

Figure 16. Demonstration of innervation of facet joints at multiple spinal levels. The medial branch nerves are finer than a fine pencil point and are highly vulnerable to stretch injury from flexion-hyperextension type trauma. Once these nerves are stretched, healing may not be effective, resulting in a chronic pain syndrome.

Here is a fundamental point in the entire field of chronic pain management. There are patients who have painful knees or shoulders without any major structural abnormalities on MRI. Our first impulse in medicine is to label the patient a malingerer, fraud, or drug seeker because of the lack of objective evidence. This is quite unfair in many cases. There are times when the absence of a meaningful, positive diagnostic test does not mean that there is absence of pain.

This principle that I am describing exists throughout the body. If a patient complaining of knee pain sustained an injury to any of the nerves responsible for the sensory innervation of the knee, chronic pain similar to pain sustained in an injury to the ligaments, cartilage, or bones of the knee will result. Most peripheral nerves (outside the CNS) can only perform specific functions, sense their environment, determine position relative to the rest of the body, and contract a muscle. (There are also autonomic sensory nerves that have other functions such as temperature regulation, influence over function of the internal organs, and modulation of the endocrine system. Damage to these nerves can also cause chronic pain syndromes such as diabetic neuropathy.) An injured peripheral nerve can respond only two ways: yell in pain to the brain or cause the muscles associated with it to contract. That is why muscle spasm frequently accompanies pain. **Therefore, chronic joint pain** *anywhere in the body* **can be due either to frank injury to the joint or due to injury to a nerve that gives sensation to that joint**. This concept is foreign to many if not most doctors, and the failure to recognize joint pain from nerve injury is responsible for much unnecessary surgery, and many frustrated patients following unsuccessful and unnecessary surgery. It makes no sense to operate on a minor structural problem when the cause of pain is a damaged nerve.

One last point requires our consideration. If the disc herniation does not necessarily indicate a source of pain, is there any value to performing the MRI of the spine? The answer is yes for at least two reasons. First, we always want to rule out a mass or lesion of the spine as a cause of pain, and second, because the herniated disc, while a relatively inert material (meaning that it has no blood supply and its contents likely do not cause inflammation of the nerve roots), gives an excellent indication of the site of injury following high-velocity trauma. This is due to the fact that in flexion-hyperextension injuries the disc gets pinched and compressed in flexion and "blows out" posteriorly, sometimes contacting the nerve root,and then in hyperextension the facet joints become compressed and damaged at the same spinal level (figure 17). Things are not always how they appear; therefore, I contend that in cases of high-velocity trauma, a herniated disc is in many cases not the cause of pain, but rather the *marker* of the spinal level of injury. I am hoping that this point of view will change the way that clinicians interpret MRIs showing herniated discs.

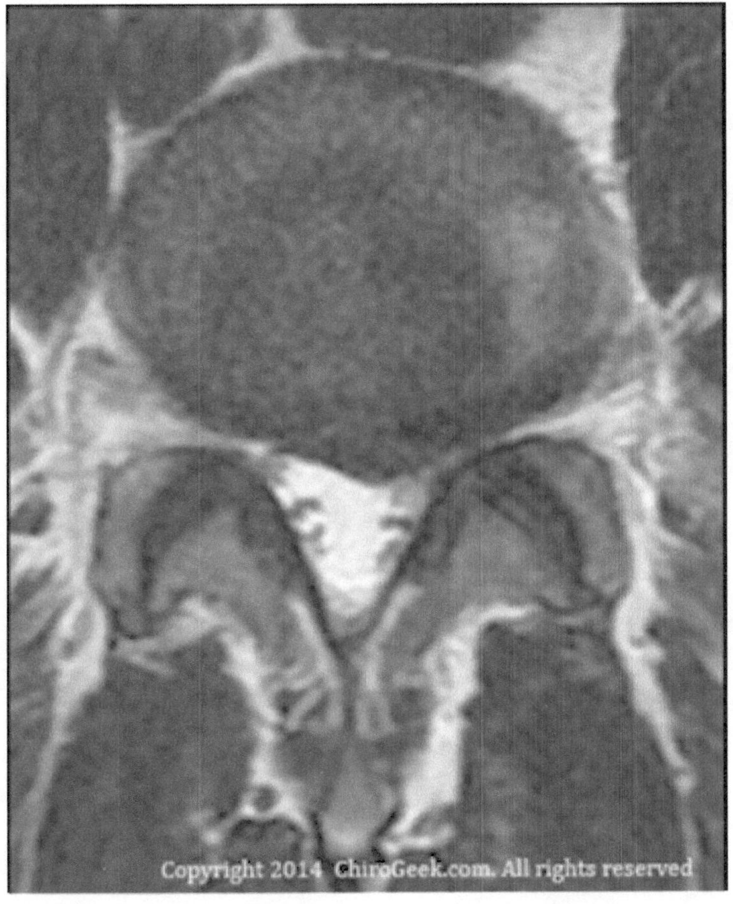

Figure 17. Radiograph of bulging lumbar disc AND bilateral facet joint inflammation. Looking at the MRI alone and not knowing the patient history and physical exam, it is impossible to determine the cause of pain.

If a patient *never* gets a proper diagnosis in terms of mechanism and causation of injury, there is almost no chance of seeing a change in condition. Proper evaluation and then treatment are the most essential services that the pain-management specialist can provide. If chronic pain patients are not properly diagnosed, how can we blame them for drug-seeking behavior and undergoing inappropriate surgeries? They only want to feel better. *Reinterpreting the meaning of a herniated disc on the MRI* will allow for more realistic diagnostic possibilities in treatment of chronic back pain.

In this chapter, you have learned the following:

- The two mechanisms by which joints can cause the sensation of pain

- The two main responses that a sensory nerve can have when there is nerve damage

- The distinction between facet arthropathy and facet syndrome

- That herniated discs are markers for the area of injury to the spine, rather than generators of pain

Chapter 5

Treatment of Injured Facet and Sacroiliac Joints

Quieting Painful Joints

Armed with greater clarity with respect to the causes of chronic pain, therapeutic options become clearer. Based on my multiple observations, I am confident that nerve injury is involved in the vast majority of chronic pain cases. This is the reason we are unsuccessful in diagnosing and treating these conditions. Ironically, despite all the advances in medicine, the one area of diagnostic imaging and testing that lags behind all the others is that which pertains to the peripheral nervous system. There is currently no specific, reliable way to image damaged peripheral nerves. Damage to the peripheral nerves is known to cause changes in the central nervous system, which have the potential to set up a vicious cycle of chronic pain.

The EMG (electromyogram) test is a neurophysiological test mainly used to diagnose neuromuscular disorders. One of the main functions of peripheral nerves is to cause muscle contraction. EMG is an excellent test for diagnosing neuromuscular and nerve conduction disorders. Unfortunately, the EMG is not a good test for sensory or painful disorders due to the different characteristics of sensory and motor nerves. While

EMG can give an *indication* of the integrity and function of some sensory nerves, since sensory nerves often travel in a bundle with motor nerves, overall these tests are overread in my experience, and many times show no abnormality when there is a clear injury to a sensory nerve. The interpretation of the EMG with regard to painful nerve disorders can be likened to attempting to paint a portrait from a silhouette; there are just not enough specific details to paint a complete picture. Unfortunately, this test, in many cases, gives another data point that in many cases is challenging to interpret since it is not a reliable, verifiable test for the smaller sensory nerves. Is there any evidence that injury to the facet joints is responsible for the perpetuation of chronic neck and LBP? In most cases involving chronic pain, it is difficult to perform randomized clinical trials on patients because of the necessity of comparing actual treatments to nontherapeutic treatments. There are ethical and moral issues with provision of sham procedures to these individuals. There may be emotional and cognitive issues that cloud a patient's ability to report the results of a procedure. Sometimes even the hope that a treatment will be helpful produces a positive effect known as the *placebo effect*. In general, the best available evidence is based on patient responses to actual treatment, which will vary from doctor to doctor. The most useful generalization is that a correct and proper diagnosis allows for the possibility of effective treatment.

You may remember that there are two conditions associated with painful facet joints. One is known as *facet arthropathy*, where the facet joint is damaged by arthritis, and the other is *facet syndrome*, where only the nerve that innervates the facet joint is damaged.

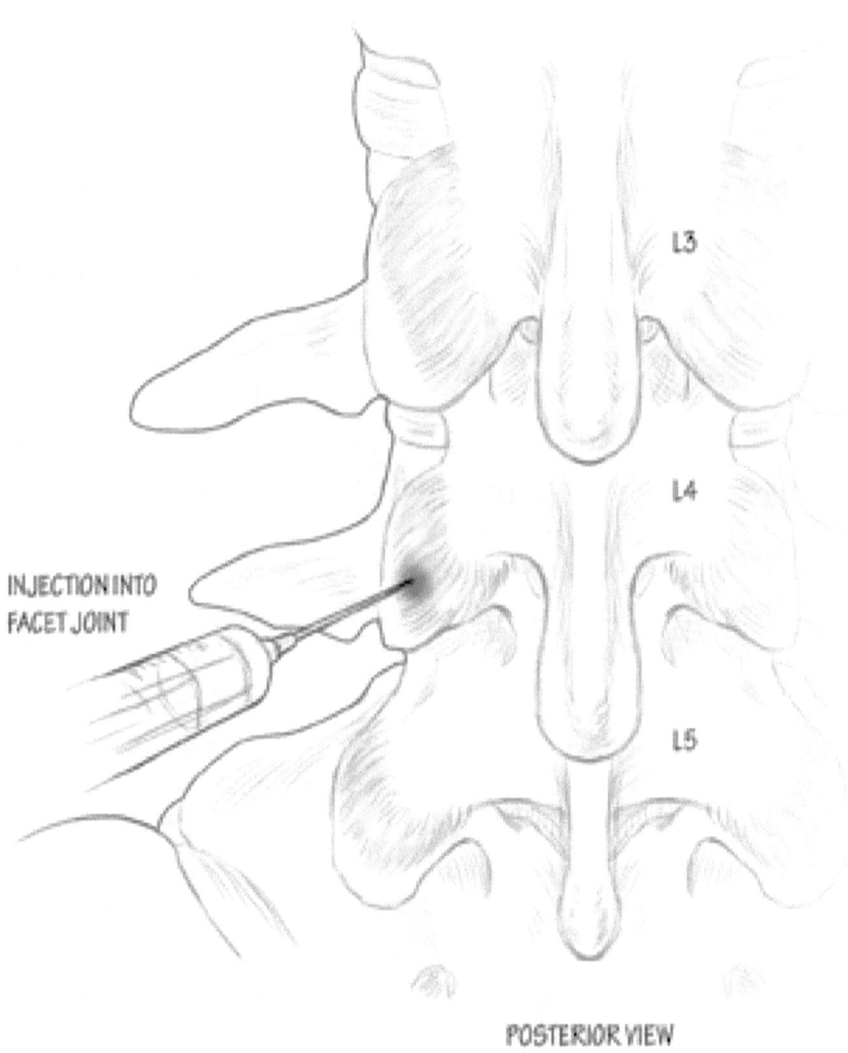

Figure 18. Injection of steroid and local anesthetic in to facet joint performed under fluoroscopy.

These conditions both produce similar symptoms and are best diagnosed by placing local anesthetic into the area suspected to be the cause of pain.

There are two types of injection that are used to diagnose and treat injury to the facet joint. The first is injection of the facet joint(s). This is not much different from injection of any major joint, such as the knee or shoulder. The facet joint injection (figure 18) is performed when the source of pain is the facet joint itself, and this determination is made upon seeing thickening of the joint or fluid in the joint (from facet arthropathy) on MRI. Clinically, patients with facet arthropathy are indistinguishable from those with facet syndrome. In some cases, just treating the area of arthritis with local anesthetic and steroids markedly diminishes the pain of arthritis. The second type of injection is the medial branch block (figure 19), which is directed *toward the nerve* that innervates the facet joint. In cases of facet syndrome, MRI findings are negative with respect to the facet joints (although there may be herniated or bulging discs) due to the fact that there is no frank injury to the joints, *but rather the damage is to the nerves that innervate the facet joints, which is not visible or detectable on any radiological or physiological study* (such as x-ray, CT scan, MRI, or EMG). The value of both of these procedures is that they are diagnostic tests of the integrity of the facet joint, its innervation, and its likelihood of being the generator of chronic pain. In most patients, there is a period of relief following these injections (if performed properly) of a few days to several weeks, as well as increased range of motion (ability to turn or bend) in the affected area. In many cases, the pain will return in a period of days or weeks following the procedure. The value of the procedure is that the exact cause of the pain has become apparent, and the next step is a procedure called radiofrequency ablation, RFA, which provides prolonged periods of relief.

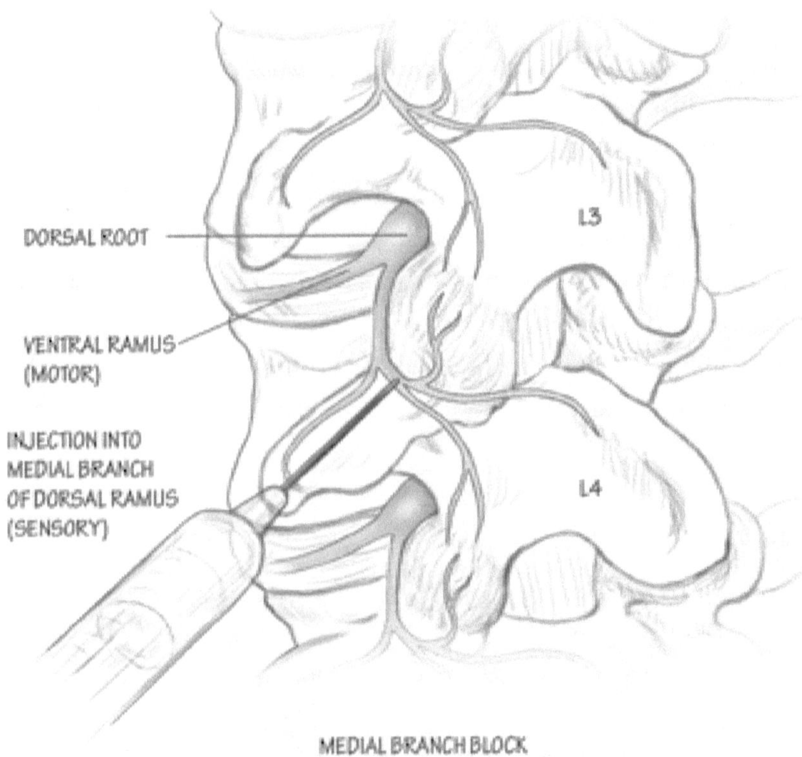

Figure 19. Medial branch block. As opposed to placing medication directly in the facet joint, medication is placed near the nerve that innervates the facet joint, similar to the nerve block you receive at the dentist. This block is most useful when the nerve to the facet joint is thought to have sustained damage rather than the facet joint itself. In cases where the medial nerve is damaged, the facet joint may appear normal, and the intervertebral disc may appear to be either normal or abnormal depending upon the forces involved in the trauma.

RFA or radiofrequency ablation (figures 20A and 20B) is a procedure in which small sensory nerves can be interrupted by a specialized needle that has a heating element at its tip. Once the needle has been placed in appropriate position under fluoroscopy, away from the nerve roots that we do not wish to destroy but close to the medial branches (we test this on the patient to be certain of proper positioning), the tip of the needle is heated to 80 degrees Celsius for a period of ninety seconds. This causes interruption of the medial nerve that travels to the facet joint for a period of twelve to eighteen months, thus diminishing the chronic pain felt in the painful joint to a significant degree. This pain may return after a year because of the regeneration of the nerves that had been heated. This procedure enables the patient, after a brief period of healing, to have increased mobility and decreased reliance on pain medicines in many cases.

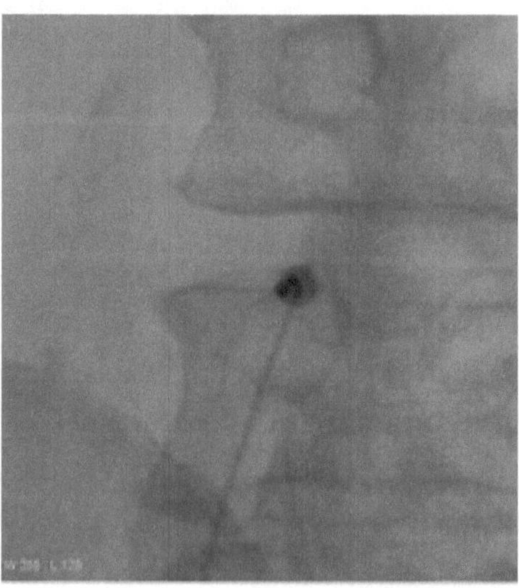

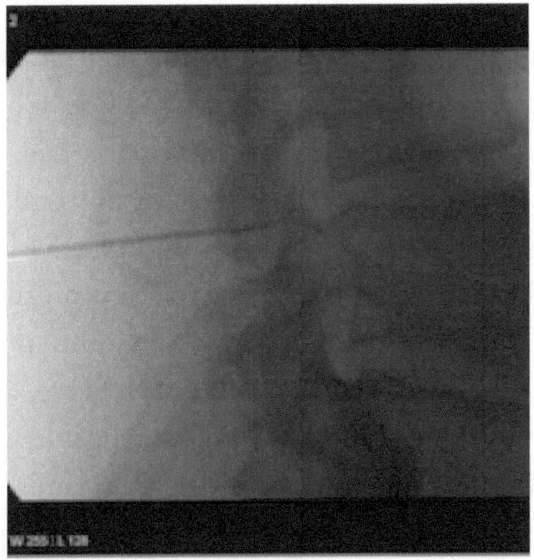

Figure 20. Radiofrequency ablation, oblique view (top) and lateral view (bottom). RFA is useful to treat both the chronic pain associated with facet joint arthritis, and also for treatment of injury to the medial branch nerve that has become injured. Since in either case it is the medial branch nerve (figure 20A and 20B) that is transmitting pain impulses to the spine and brain, interrupting the medial branch nerve with RFA will successfully treat either facet arthropathy or facet syndrome.

Case Study 2

A fifty-six-year-old man fell down a flight of stairs because he slipped on a skateboard that had been left at the top of the landing. He sustained injuries to his right hip and low back in the fall. He now complains of pain and burning sensation radiating down the side of his right leg, worst at night. His sleep is disturbed by the back pain, and there is low back stiffness each morning upon awakening. On physical examination, he was found to have pain to palpation of the right L4-S1 facet joints as well as positive right Patrick test, a test that puts stress on the sacroiliac joint, pain with light pressure of the right sacroiliac joint, and pain with light pressure of the right lateral femoral cutaneous nerve, a nerve that gives sensation to the outer thigh, above the inguinal ligament, which connects the front of the pelvis to the thighbone. There was mild numbness of the lateral right leg and decreased extension of the lumbar spine. MRI of the lumbar spine showed bulging discs at L4-L5 and L5-S1. The patient was treated with Neurontin and Motrin, but the back and leg pain persisted. Right lumbar medial branch block, which temporarily freezes the lower lumbar facet joints, was performed with good relief of low back pain and increased range of motion for six days. Then the pain returned. RFA was performed at the L4, L5, and S1 medial branches, and after an initial period of soreness, the low back pain diminished by 50 percent. After five weeks, the patient stated that there was still significant low back pain on the right side as well as continuing right leg pain and numbness. Physical exam failed to show any pain at the L4-L5, L5-S1 facet joints, but there was still pain at the right SI joint and at the right lateral femoral cutaneous nerve. The patient was reassured that when the remaining sources of pain from the SI joint and the lateral femoral cutaneous nerve were treated, he would continue to improve.

There are cases in which I will resolve the primary pain problem and the patient will continue to complain of pain. In the past, I would tell the patient that we had done the best that we could and discharge the patient—or, worse, send the patient for surgery. As I began to understand the issues involved in treating chronic pain, I realized that once one area of the neck or back had diminished painful sensation, adjacent areas, or sometimes even areas somewhat distant from the original pain, might begin to be perceived as a source of pain. This is because our processing mechanism in the spine is usually barraged by the more intense pain signal (the stronger pain), and less intense pain messages are muted. Once the stronger pain stimulus is blunted, the less intense pain stimulus will be processed because it becomes more noticeable. Just as cars must go through a tollbooth one by one, painful impulses are processed individually, with the worst pain receiving the most attention and emotional response. Often, when treatment is incomplete, in the sense that not all of the generators of pain have been treated, it is appropriate not to blame the patient but rather to reexamine the patient and search for additional painful joints or nerves that formerly were overshadowed by the more severe pain, which, once treated, will allow for recognition of other painful areas. Viewed in this context, it is easy to understand why pain patients and doctors are frequently at odds with each other, why there is such confusion and frustration on the part of patients and doctors, and why society looks askance at people suffering with chronic pain.

Another potential source of chronic low back pain is the sacroiliac joints. These joints can be injured by high-velocity trauma, a combination of vertical compression and rapid rotation, (lifting a heavy object and twisting), or falling on the backside. The sacroiliac joints can also become arthritic from autoimmune disorders such as ankylosing spondylitis, rheumatoid arthritis, psoriatic arthritis, ulcerative colitis, and sarcoidosis and also certain infections such as tuberculosis and gonorrhea. The sacroiliac joint helps transfer the weight of the upper body to the pelvis and lower extremities. The SI joint is irregularly shaped and moves minimally, only 2–4 mm in any direction. The SI joints act to tilt the pelvis so as to keep the center of gravity slightly in front of the spine during walking and standing. (See figure 21.)

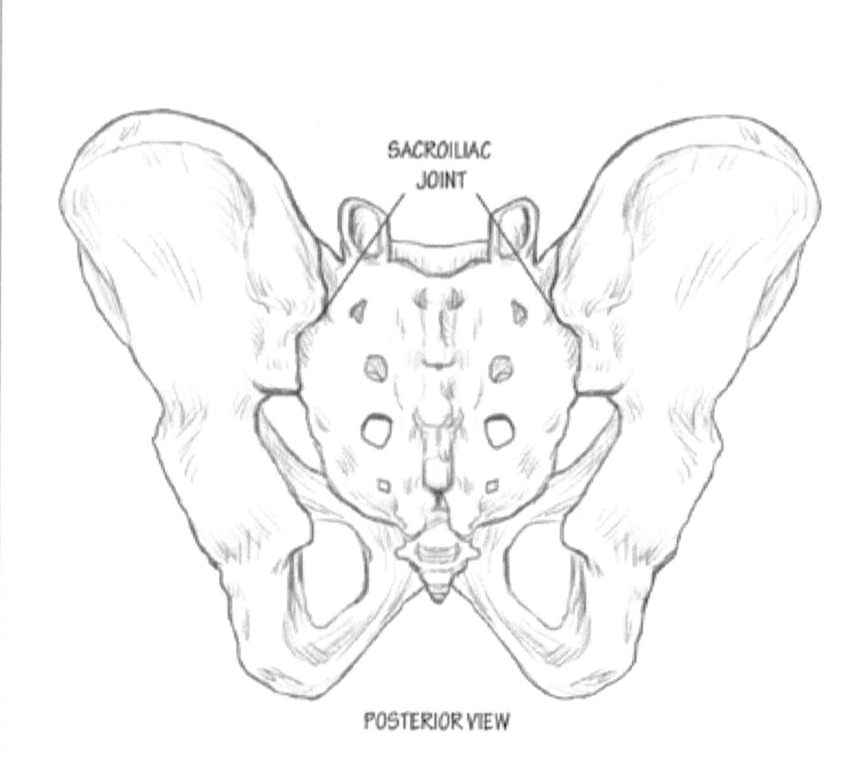

Figure 21. Anatomy of sacroiliac joints, posterior view

By virtue of their position at the junction of the spine and pelvis, the SI joints are vulnerable to traumatic injury. For reasons that are unclear, they are also targets for inflammation by the aforementioned diseases and infectious agents. In many cases, the pain will radiate to the buttock on the side of the injured SI joint. The Patrick test, in which the sacroiliac joint is stressed, is a useful method for diagnosing SI joint pain (figure 22). In some cases, the SI joint will respond to injection with steroid and local anesthetic, but in many cases the relief is short-lived. In some instances, RFA of the nerves that innervate the SI joint (S1-S4 medial branches) will help relieve some of the pain. SI joint pain may not be easily detectable if other causes of low back pain exist simultaneously, because L4-L5, L5-S1 herniated discs can cause sacroiliac joint pain and also because of the complexities of the nervous system in processing multiple sensations of pain simultaneously, as alluded to earlier.

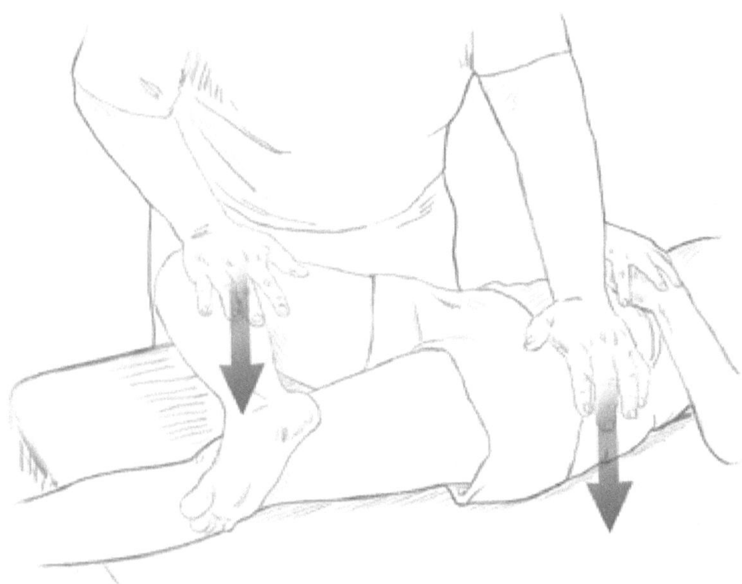

Figure 22. Patrick test for assessing whether sacroiliac joint is responsible for back pain.

Our bones are connected by ligaments, tendons, joints, and other soft tissues. In high-velocity injuries, it is not uncommon for forces to act on adjacent tissues that move in unison and become injured at the same time. For example, both the lower lumbar facet joints and the SI joints, which have attachments to both the pelvis and spine, can become injured in the same accident. In addition, because the hip is also attached to the pelvis by ligamentous attachments, the nerve that is in close proximity to the hip, the lateral femoral cutaneous nerve, which provides sensation to the outer thigh, and the femoral nerve, which provides sensation to the inner thigh, can be injured in trauma involving the lower pelvis. I like to think of these injuries that cluster together as symptom complexes. This will be discussed in greater length in Chapter 7.

In this chapter, you have learned the following:

- The limited role of EMG in diagnosis of chronic neck and back pain.

- The similarities and differences of facet arthropathy and facet syndrome.

- Why chronic painful facet joints fit the definition of chronic pain.

- Diagnostic testing and therapeutic strategies for painful facet joints.

Chapter 6

Nerve Injury in the Spine and the Rest of the Body

Nerves Don't Like to Be Irritated

I have introduced a number of concepts that are not traditionally taught in medical school. The reason that these radical ideas are necessary is that traditional medicine continues to disappoint and fail a large number of chronic pain sufferers. Injuries to nerves need to be considered from the perspective of whether the nerve injury is central (brain or spine) or peripheral in nature, and whether somatic or autonomic in nature. It is always difficult to differentiate between central and peripheral (in the limb). This task is confusing because any peripheral nerve injury has aspects of a central nervous system injury, because of their intimate association. If one suffers a traumatic amputation of a limb, one cut edge of the nerves of the amputated limb is still attached to the spinal cord and brain. There are definite changes that occur in the spinal cord and brain due to the peripheral nerve injury. The converse can also be true. Sometimes central nerve injuries can be felt in the periphery. An example of this occurs in some cases of multiple sclerosis, when a nerve damage due to *demyelination* (loss of insulation of a nerve) in the brain can cause sensation of nerve pain in the extremities. Since nerve tissue is alive and generates electrical impulses, there are many chronic diseases (such as diabetes, postherpetic neuralgia, or reflex sympathetic dystrophy) and injuries that cause chronic pain symptoms.

For purposes of diagnosis and treatment, it is most useful to know if pain is predominantly central or peripheral. In some cases, quieting a peripheral nerve injury will also cause the corresponding terminals in the brain to become quiescent.[14]

The area where sensations from outside the spine enter the central nervous system is in the area of the nerve root and a collection of cell nuclei, the part of the nerve cell that contains its genetic material, known as the *dorsal root ganglion*. The nerves branch out from the nerve root, in some cases becoming efferent nerves that supply muscles, in other cases becoming afferent nerves bringing sensation from the periphery to the spine and brain, and in many cases becoming mixed afferent and efferent nerves, like a two-lane highway of impulses running in opposite directions (figure 23).

---

14   Chronic Post-Herpetic Neuropathy Pain Modulation by Lidoderm Patch. Apkarianlab.northwestern.edu/publications/SFN 2004 New PHN post.pd.

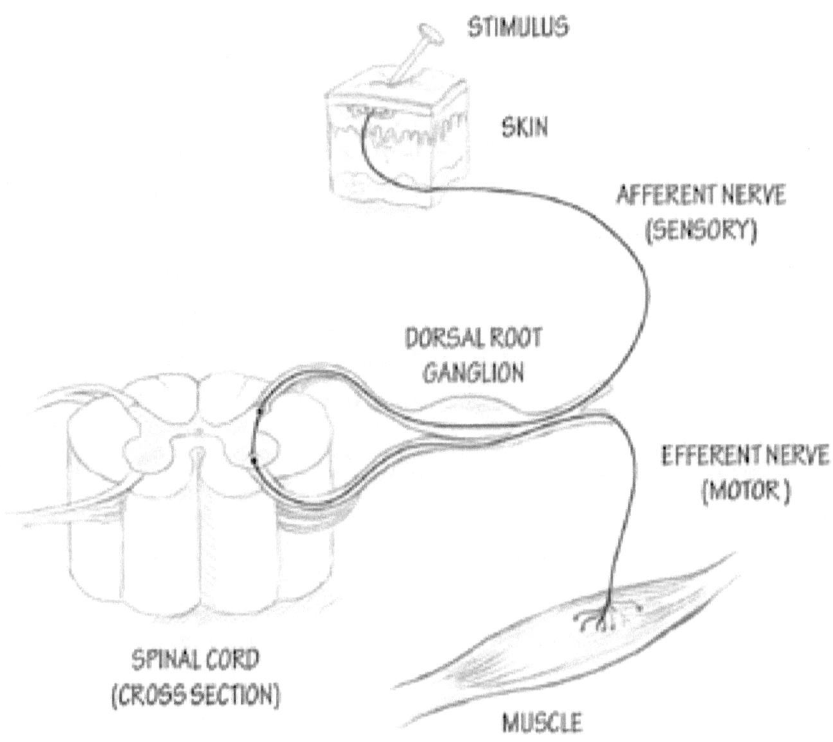

Figure 23. Sensory and motor impulse transmission in the somatic system.

Sensory transmission in many cases begins at the skin. We sense temperature, pressure, position, vibration, noxious stimuli, and pain at millions of points along the shallow and deeper levels of the skin. There is so much information coming in from the peripheral environment to be processed by the central nervous system that a major function of the brain and spinal cord is to filter out irrelevant information. Imagine sitting on a chair that rolls; there is pressure on your back and buttocks where your body contacts the chair, there is the issue of balance should you choose to recline in the chair, and also possible vibration if the ball bearings need grease, and finally there are the forces of placing your feet on the floor and extending your knees and flexing your hips when you try to rise from the chair. Irrelevant stimuli and sensations rarely come into our consciousness due to the filtering function of the CNS.

The sensory and motor nerves are considered *first order nerves*. This is an anatomic description of the fact that the nerves from the periphery consist of one cell and nucleus, with the nuclei found in the dorsal root ganglion, and the first synapse or connection made within the spinal cord. From there, several more connections are made to various regions of the brain and also within the spinal cord (figure 24). For this reason, the sensory nerves that are in your toes and fingertips are some of the longest in the body. They are also the most vulnerable to fluctuations in blood supply, oxygen, and certain metabolic abnormalities, such as diabetes and toxins that affect the nervous system.

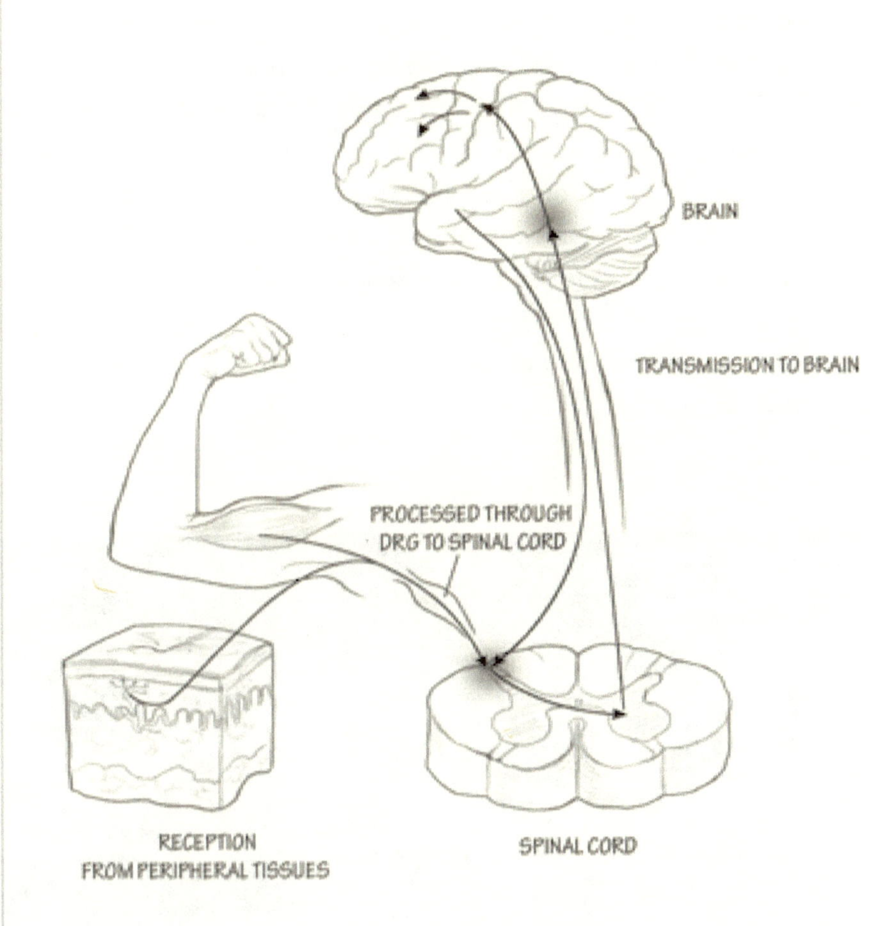

Figure 24. Transmission of painful impulses from periphery to spine and brain and back to muscle for withdrawal from noxious stimuli.

I have mentioned the consequences of a sensory nerve being cut in the case of amputation. What happens when peripheral nerves are injured by stretch, compression, or lack of oxygen? If a nerve is not severed, it can still become damaged in a fashion such that the transmission of information along the axon (long part of the nerve) is adversely affected. A nerve damaged in any of these three ways has a significant advantage over one that has been severed. The nerve that has not been cut benefits from preservation of its outer architecture, providing the framework or path for the nerve to reconstitute and regenerate. Unfortunately, the nerve grows back and regains function very slowly. A severed nerve will actually send out sprouts in order to try to find its other end (figure 25). This can contribute to development of chronic pain if the edges of severed nerves are not close together.

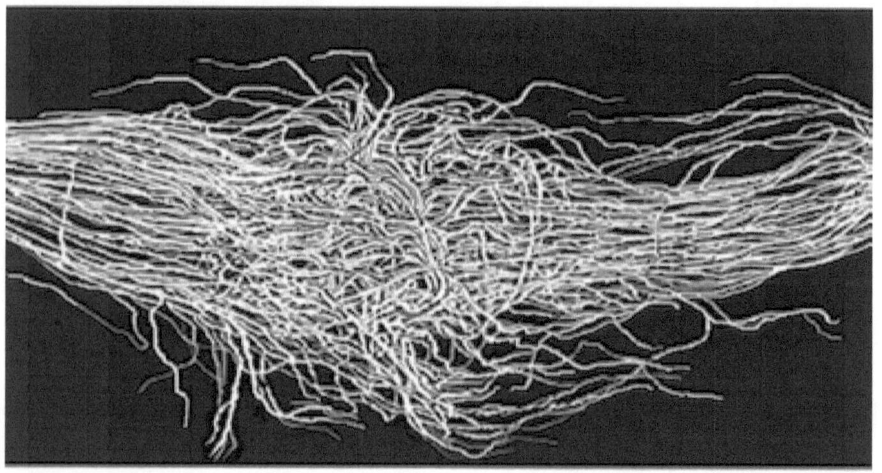

Figure 25. Damaged (severed) nerve reconstitution.

How does a nerve become stretched or compressed? The most common causes are associated with trauma. Peripheral nerves are largely tethered to the spinal cord and also connected to the tissues through which they travel. If there is an acceleration/ deceleration injury, as occurs in a motor vehicle accident (MVA), nerves can be violently and rapidly flexed and extended. A good example of this type of injury is the trauma to the small medial branch that innervates the facet joints of the spine, which was discussed earlier. The rapid, sudden motion is enough to stretch and injure the very small-caliber and delicate nerves that innervate the facet joints (figure 26). The same type of injury can occur at any of the peripheral nerves, which can be stretched or compressed depending on their location relative to the traumatic event. Surgery or fracturing a bone, such as the ankle or elbow, can cause stretch or compression injury of nerves adjacent to the point of trauma or injury. In some cases, even though a fracture is reduced or fixed, pain persists due to injury of the adjacent nerve. This sounds a lot like a description of chronic pain. Unfortunately, doctors are not taught to process information in this fashion in medical school, so it may be difficult to get a proper diagnosis.

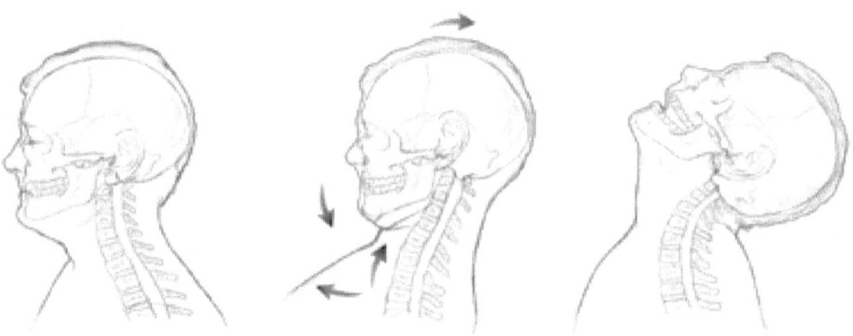

Figure 26. Flexion-hyperextension type of injury of cervical spine. Intervertebral discs, facet joints, and medial branch nerves are all vulnerable to become damaged due to forces involved.

Nerve compression can occur in several different ways. In many cases, nerves are compressed extrinsically, that is, from the outside of the body. If pressure is placed on a sensory or motor nerve for a prolonged period of time, the blood supply to the nerve can become compromised, and there can be pain and weakness in the distribution of that nerve, and in severe cases even damage to muscle tissue. This is why in surgical cases that require a tourniquet, we try not to inflate it beyond a certain pressure, and not longer than forty-five to sixty minutes.

There are many reports in the literature of the ulnar and femoral nerves being damaged either by improper positioning of the patient's body during anesthesia or from retractors compressing nerves. Anesthesiologists are particularly concerned with proper positioning to prevent compression of nerves, since patients under anesthesia are unable to report unusual sensations. There have been some cases in which the body of the surgeon or heavy instruments have come into contact with and compressed a nerve while the patient is anesthetized, resulting in nerve injury, pain, and weakness. Neuritis is a milder form of nerve damage, irritation, or inflammation, and neuropathy is a more severe form.

There can also be internal causes of nerve compression. These have also been called *tunnel syndromes*, due to the fact that nerves travel through tissue planes and are sometimes compressed and trapped in areas where ligaments or fascia, a sheath of fibrous tissue, traverse bone. The best-known tunnel syndrome is carpal tunnel syndrome in which the median nerve at the wrist is compressed by a thickened carpal ligament (figure 27). This can cause numbness, tingling, and even weakness in the palm and fingers. There are a host of tunnel syndromes, and it is important for any health care professional treating patients with pain to have a working knowledge of them all. Ligaments can be damaged and thickened from trauma, infections, and autoimmune diseases, as well as altered metabolic states such as diabetes, hyperthyroidism, and pregnancy. The lateral femoral cutaneous nerve can be compressed in overweight people due to pressure from the fat and the femoral ligament; this is called *meralgia paresthetica.*

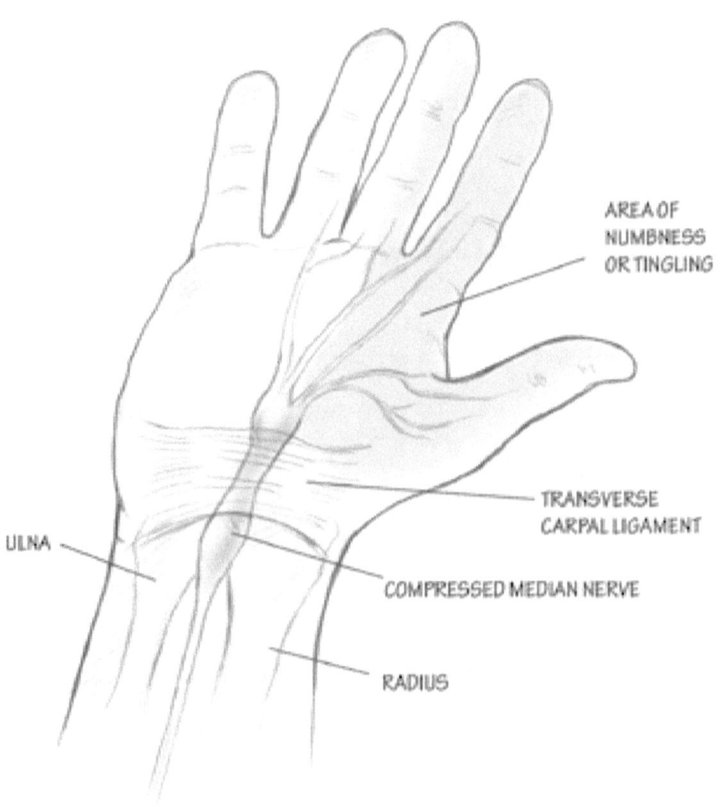

Figure 27. Development of tunnel syndrome generally involves compression of the median nerve at the wrist by the carpal ligament. This is a very common cause of nerve compression in many cases treated by severing the carpal ligament. It is not uncommon for people to exercise, sleep, or rest (like watching a movie) with a nerve inadvertently hyperextended causing stretch and injury, especially involving the nerves of the hands (figure 28). In most cases the architecture of the axon is well-preserved and in only the most extreme cases is there permanent or long-standing pain, numbness, or weakness due to permanent damage to the axons.

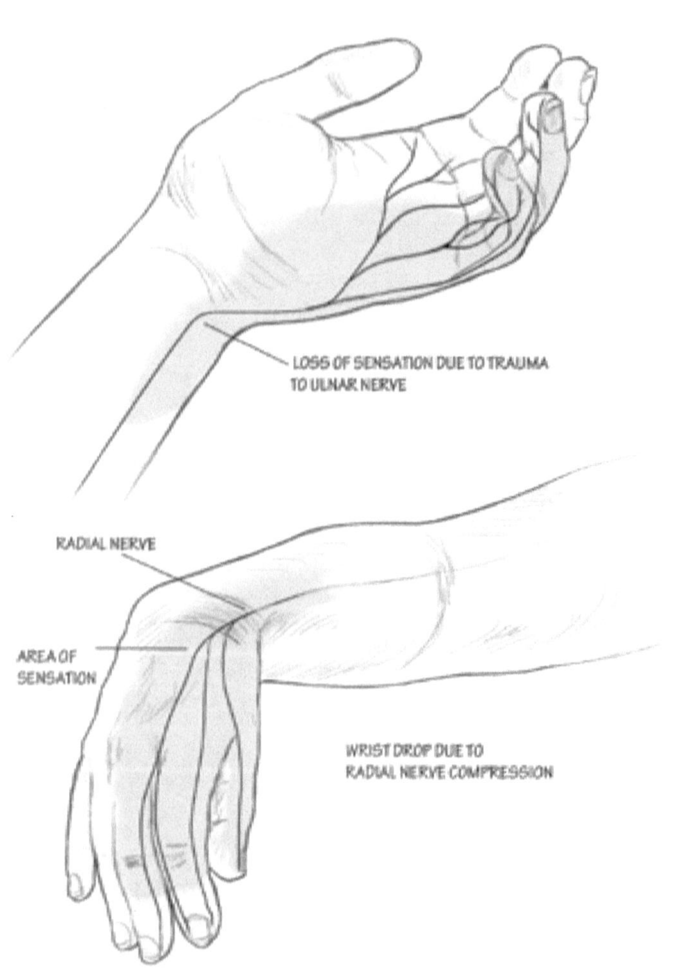

Figure 28. Stretch injury or compression injury to nerves can cause weakness, tingling, and numbness in the distribution of affect nerve.

On occasion, surgical intervention is required to cut or weaken the thickened ligament so that pressure is removed from the nerve. I have found in many cases of nerve injury involving the shoulders, hands, elbows, ankles, knees, and hips that just by placing steroid medication and local anesthetic in the area of a compressed peripheral nerve, there is almost immediate relief, thus establishing a diagnosis, and in many cases that relief can be sustained for many months. These patients whose pain essentially emanates from compression of a nerve also meet the criteria for the diagnosis of chronic pain. To reiterate, in many cases of chronic pain, there is a nerve that has sustained some type of insult or injury. This seems so simple to understand, yet it is not universally recognized. Just as when you bring your new car in for repair, if the sensor that relates to the defective or damaged part is not activated, then there is no evidence of a problem. There are rare exceptions where the sensors are "broken," such as people born with sensory nerves that do not sense pain, or damage to small nerve fibers from diabetes or TB that can cause diminished perception of pain.

Generally, doctors have been trained to look for radicular signs or *radiculopathy*, especially in patients with herniated discs or space occupying lesions of the spine such as tumors or abscesses (figure 29). We always want to treat a compressed nerve root, which results in radiculopathy in order to relieve any pressure that may be causing weakness, numbness, or tingling in a dermatome. A *dermatome* is a map of the area or territory innervated by each nerve root as it emanates from the spine (figure 30). I was always puzzled when patients would have pain and weakness in some parts of the dermatome but not others. In the past, we reasoned that not all fibers of a nerve root were being compressed by a herniated disc, and therefore, for example, only the fibers that innervate the knee and not the hip were affected. While this may be true, it takes tremendous sleight of hand (to mix metaphors) for a nerve root to be partially affected by compression at only one specific anatomical region. I like to examine each peripheral sensory nerve, especially at points of injury, areas that nerves can be compressed against bone, and areas known to be susceptible to stretch injury or tunnel syndromes. I am always amazed at the extent and number of peripheral nerve injuries that I am able to discover and that are responsible for chronic pain.

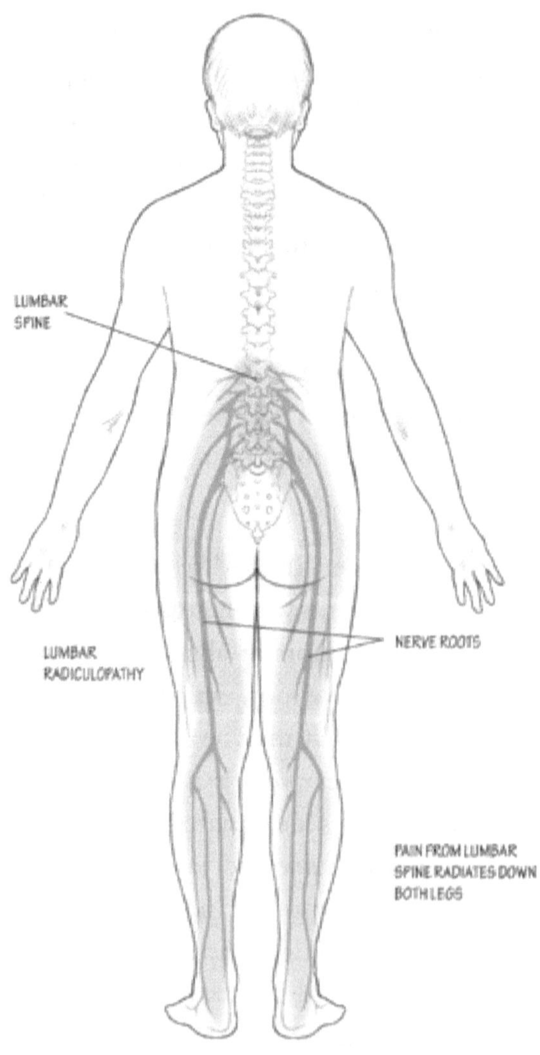

Figure 29. Radiculopathy in the lower extremities Pain, weakness or numbness travels from area of low back or hip down to foot.

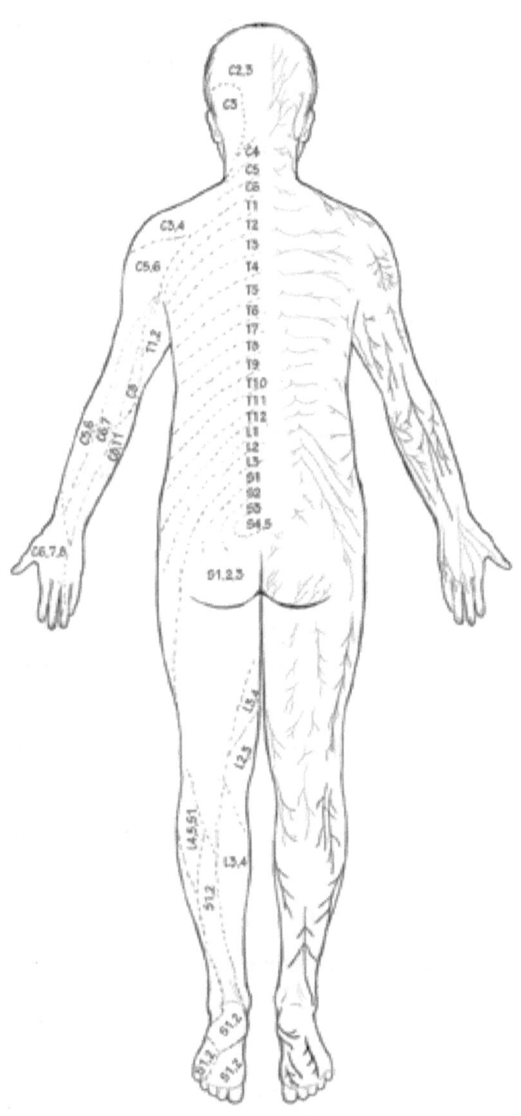

Figure 30. Dermatomal map of the body from posterior view

I do not mean to say that radiculopathy is not an important cause of pain. Pain that runs from the neck down the arm and into the fingers is almost always radicular in nature. Similarly, this is true for low back pain that radiates from the buttock to the thigh, then the calf and foot. The problem is that clinical tests that show signs of irritation of nerve roots are often negative and frequently misinterpreted. For example, the straight leg raising test is supposed to demonstrate radiculopathy by causing pain to travel down the leg by stretching the nerve root. In many cases, the patient has pain with lifting the leg from hamstring tightness or sacroiliac joint irritation. This does cause pain, but without pain radiating down the *entire* arm or leg, it cannot therefore be interpreted as an indication of radiculopathy. (See figure 14.)

Radicular pain by itself is not an indication for surgery, but if there is associated weakness in the affected limb of the muscles that emanate from the nerve root that is compressed, surgery is indicated, since prolonged pressure on a motor nerve can cause significant long-lasting weakness or atrophy.

The term *radiculitis* indicates that there is inflammation in the affected nerve root causing pain but little or no weakness in the extremity. This concept fits well with the theory that a torn annulus can cause leakage of the inner "toxic" disc material on the nerve root. This should result in pain that radiates in the affected dermatome, and treatment with epidural steroid injection should help to relieve the inflammation almost immediately. There is evidence that inflammatory chemicals are present near discs that have herniated. It is not clear whether the inflammation is due to the torn annulus and leakage of disc material or due to some other factor such as inflammation at the nearby facet joints. It is known that the posteriorly located facet joints have an adequate blood supply, whereas the intervertebral discs do not have any significant blood supply, and perhaps the inflammatory chemicals that result from injury are more easily transported by the bloodstream to areas adjacent to facet joints, and they may then diffuse or leak to the area of the nearby disc.

Some physicians have sought to prove the existence of torn discs by placing dye in the center of the discs. This test is known as discography. Usually the affected disc(s) and one normal adjacent disc (as a control) are tested. Patients are awake during this test and are able to confirm whether increasing pressure in the disc causes pain. If there is pain with pressure from dye injection, this is known as a concordant disc (figure 31). Following placement of the dye, a CT scan of the spine is performed, which is able to show areas of dye leakage, which indicate a torn annulus.

In recent years, because of the concept that small changes in disc volume create large changes in pressure on nerve roots, percutaneous discectomy has emerged as an effective treatment for painful herniated discs. This minimally invasive procedure cauterizes a small amount of the inner nucleus pulposis substance called glycoproteins, thus causing a significant decrease in pressure exerted by the outer annulus fibrosis on nerve roots. This procedure is beneficial because it preserves the architecture of the discs, while relieving pain. It is performed via a specialized needle which cauterizes the inner disc, causing decrease in pressure exerted on the nerve root by herniated disc material, thus significantly reducing rehabilitation and recovery times.

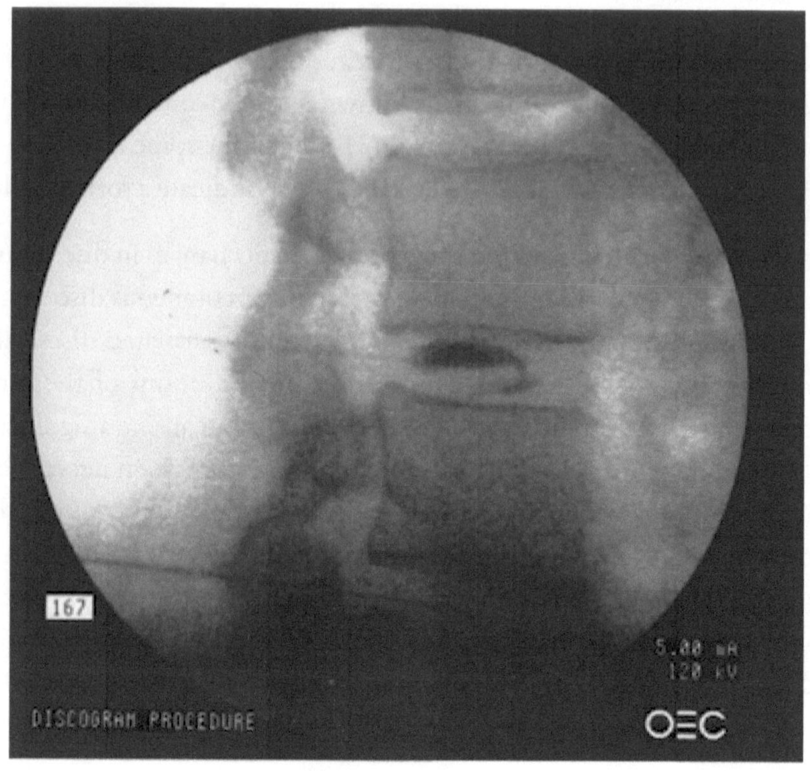

Figure 31. Discogram of lower lumbar segmental discs.

The inner disc material is relatively inert, and I don't feel that the nucleus pulposis material is toxic to nerve roots. In my opinion most bulging and herniated discs are *markers of damage to the spinal column, and only in some cases are generators of ongoing pain*. It is difficult to recommend disc surgery in a case where there is pain, but also a bulging disc that is not in contact with the spine or nerve root and in the absence of sensory or motor abnormalities. It would seem more prudent to look at other causes of back pain such as sacroiliac or facet joints as generators of pain in such a case.

While it is clear that there are cases of disc herniation and radiculopathy that may require urgent treatment, these are in the minority of circumstances. I believe that there are many more cases that peripheral nerves have been injured by compression or stretch injury, in high-velocity trauma. This would include motor vehicle accidents, sports injuries, and slip and falls. There is no good diagnostic test as of today to locate and image a damaged nerve that is of small caliber. A doctor sometimes has to use his or her imagination to fill in the missing gaps of information, rather than blaming the patient for information that does not perfectly fit together. Many clinicians make the error of assuming that pain radiating to an extremity is always from irritation of a nerve root. This is not the case. If a nerve such as the lateral femoral cutaneous nerve is stretched and injured in an accident, there will be pain and tingling down the outside or lateral leg. If the femoral nerve is damaged in the area of the groin, which can happen if the steering wheel pushes into the pelvic area, there will be pain and possibly sensory abnormality in the inner thigh area. If careful examination of the individual peripheral nerves is not carried out, these pains can be mistakenly interpreted as radiculopathy. Pseudo-radiculopathy occurs when peripheral nerve injuries are erroneously diagnosed as radicular nerve injuries. This is not a small point, because when examining nerves and assessing the extent of any injury, we are also making inferences as to the extent and location of the damage that has occurred, and these decisions will shape a treatment plan. If we make incorrect inferences, then the diagnosis is likely to be wrong and the treatment rendered ineffective.

Due to the fact that the peripheral nerves are tethered to the spine, in many cases of traumatic injury, several injuries can commonly be seen in clusters that are not radicular in nature, or at least cannot be understood as following a radicular pattern. This concept will be discussed in the next chapter.

In this chapter, you have learned the following:

- The difficulties in describing and classifying peripheral and central nerve injuries

- Two mechanical mechanisms of sensory nerve injury in a nonsevered nerve

- Definitions of neuropathy, radiculopathy, radiculitis, and pseudo-radiculopathy

- The concept of dermatome

- The role of discography as a diagnostic test for back and neck pain.

Chapter 7

Symptom Complexes or Complex Symptoms

Why Some Headaches Don't Go Away

I am certain that if you are a chronic pain sufferer you have been closely following my ideas, and at this point you probably know more about chronic pain than I did when I got my M.D. degree in 1984, from Mount Sinai. Speaking of Mount Sinai, even Moses was known to drop a tablet now and then; nobody is perfect, and my feeling has always been that learning is a lifelong process.

Let's take a broader view to create a more meaningful picture of why you hurt. Understand that while I have taken a systematic approach that may be novel, my approach will help a large group of those patients who share the characteristics I have described.

I have stressed the importance of understanding the relationship between form and function. It does not matter whether you believe in evolution or creationism or some combination of the two. The fact is that our anatomy is not just some random collection of features. We are designed to walk upright, have a sense of balance, keep our center of gravity in front of us most of the time, have the ability to sense the environment both internally and externally, and respond to a variety of conditions whether threatening or nonthreatening. The way that we are constructed significantly influences the ways that we interact with our environment. It is no different regarding the complex physical, behavioral, and social interactions involving chronic pain.

Because of the many anatomic connections of our bodies, outer forces that act on our bodies generally do not affect individual structures. When you break your ankle, you do not only damage the bone there is also trauma to the ligaments, blood vessels, lymphatics and nerves that surround the broken bone. This is true for surgery as well. When your hernia is fixed, the surgeon goes through layers of skin, fat, and connective tissue, as well as nerve fibers, blood vessels, and muscle fibers. It is easy to damage a nerve during hernia surgery, and some unfortunate people do experience chronic pain due to the nerve injury.

In a similar fashion, high-velocity trauma to the neck and low back areas of the spine can cause a series of injuries in the region of the impact and the region of the momentum from the impact. Newton's First Law states that for every force there is an equal and opposite force. If your vehicle is hit on the front end, your neck will flex forward, and the rest of your body will move forward. Upon application of the brakes, your neck will extend, and your body will slam backward. The reverse is true for rear-end collisions; the neck extends, and the body first moves back, and with application of the brake, the neck and body move forward. (See figure 26.) It is easy to understand how the joints of the spine are damaged in this scenario and also how the nerves to those joints can become stretched and damaged. But that is only the most obvious part of what has happened. When the cervical spine is injured in this fashion, there is always the possibility of fracture of one or more of the cervical vertebrae, or compromise to a vessel such as the carotid artery. The trachea and thoracic aorta could become lacerated. All these outcomes, which fortunately are rare, demand immediate medical attention and surgical intervention. In most cases, the forces are transmitted to local structures such as the thoracic spine, shoulders, arms, and hands. It is not uncommon to find stretch injury of the suprascapular nerve at the posterior shoulder, the median and ulnar nerves at the elbow, and the median nerve at the wrist. These are the most common peripheral nerve injuries that go along with neck injury, although other types of nerve injury can be seen as well. The extent and type of injury is really just a reflection of the extent and type of force that was delivered to the body at the time of injury. An astute clinician will try to work backward from the injuries in an attempt to understand the mechanism of injury. This is another example of why asking "how this happened" is at least as important as assessing "what has happened."

There are two other conditions that require special attention with cervical spine injury. The first relates to the brain. As a result of trauma to the neck in whiplash injuries, there is sometimes traumatic brain injury or post-concussion syndrome (figure 32). This can occur even in the absence of head trauma, due to shearing forces in the cranium. There can be prolonged dizziness, gait disturbance, nausea, cognitive impairment, as well as memory loss. This has received much press lately in the sports world, but it is germane to any high-velocity trauma. As you can imagine, in some cases this type of injury is debilitating and requires intensive periods of rehabilitation. Recently, there has been some indication that vitamin D[15] and hyperbaric oxygen[16] are useful in treating the symptoms of traumatic brain injury and in restoring some neural function in the brain.

---

15   A. Petraglia et al., "Stuck at the Bench: Potential Natural Neuroprotective Compounds for Concussion," www.ncbi.nih.gov.

16   R. Boussi-Gross et al., "Hyperbaric Oxygen Therapy Can Improve Post Concussion Syndrome Years after Mild Traumatic Brain Injury Randomized Prospective Trial," PLoS One 8, no. 11 (Nov 15, 2013), e79995, doi:10. 1371/journal.pone.0079995.eCollection.

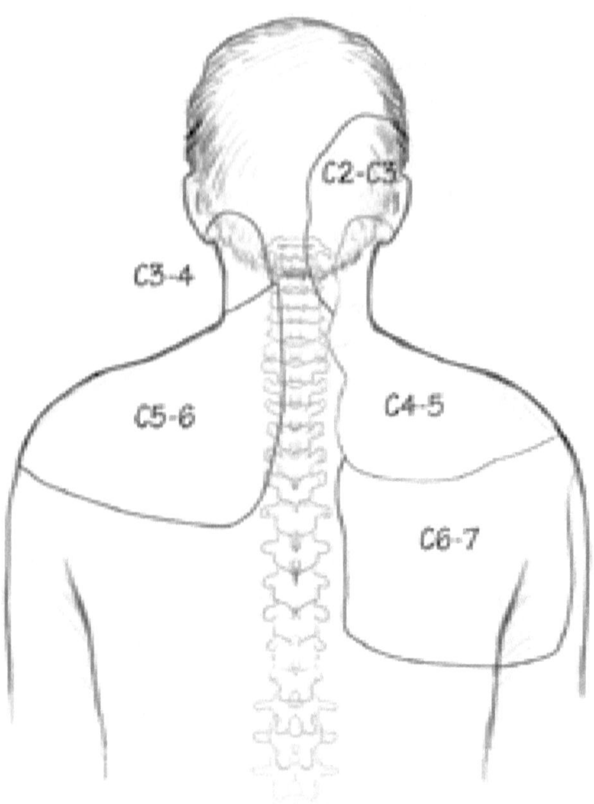

Figure 32. Map of referred pain in posterior cervical and thoracic areas from facet joint injury, by segmental level. This is not an example of radicular pain but rather pain referred from damage to facet joints. Recognizing the difference between the two is critical for making proper diagnosis and appropriate therapy.

The second condition that occurs frequently with upper cervical trauma is headache. Many patients note the onset of headache shortly after the trauma. In many cases, this subsides with time, but there are a good number of people who suffer from chronic headache following neck injury. If the cause is undetected or unsuspected, these headaches can last for many years.

Case Study 3

A fifty-three year old woman came to my office with a history of neck and shoulder pain and stiffness and weekly headaches that she had been having for the past ten years. The headaches began after a fall from a horse ten years ago, and the neck and shoulder pain began after a minor fender-bender two years ago. Chiropractic treatment gave only temporary relief. On physical exam, there was diminished range of motion of the cervical spine for extension and lateral rotation. There was pain to palpation of the bilateral upper cervical and upper thoracic facet joints or occipital nerves. MRI showed protruded discs at C3-C4 and C4-C5 with associated facet hypertrophy, meaning enlargement of the joint, at both levels. MRI of the thoracic spine was normal. The patient's headaches responded well to Topamax 25 mg three times a day. The neck pain decreased with stretch exercises and bilateral cervical and thoracic facet joint injections.

The mechanism of these headaches is related to nerve injury of the facet joints (figure 33). Along the upper cervical spine run small fibers that innervate the base of the skull to form branches of the occipital nerves. These small branches as well as the occipital nerve can become damaged in high-velocity trauma and in some cases of arthritis. Damage to these fibers causes persistent headache due to increased electrical activity in the damaged nerves. This headache is very different from migraines or tension headaches. It does not have an aura, may not be associated with muscle spasm, and is usually well localized and reproduced by pressing over the injured facet joints. These headaches respond favorably in many cases to a medication that lowers electrical activity in nerves, such as Topamax, which is being used by neurologists frequently to treat headache.

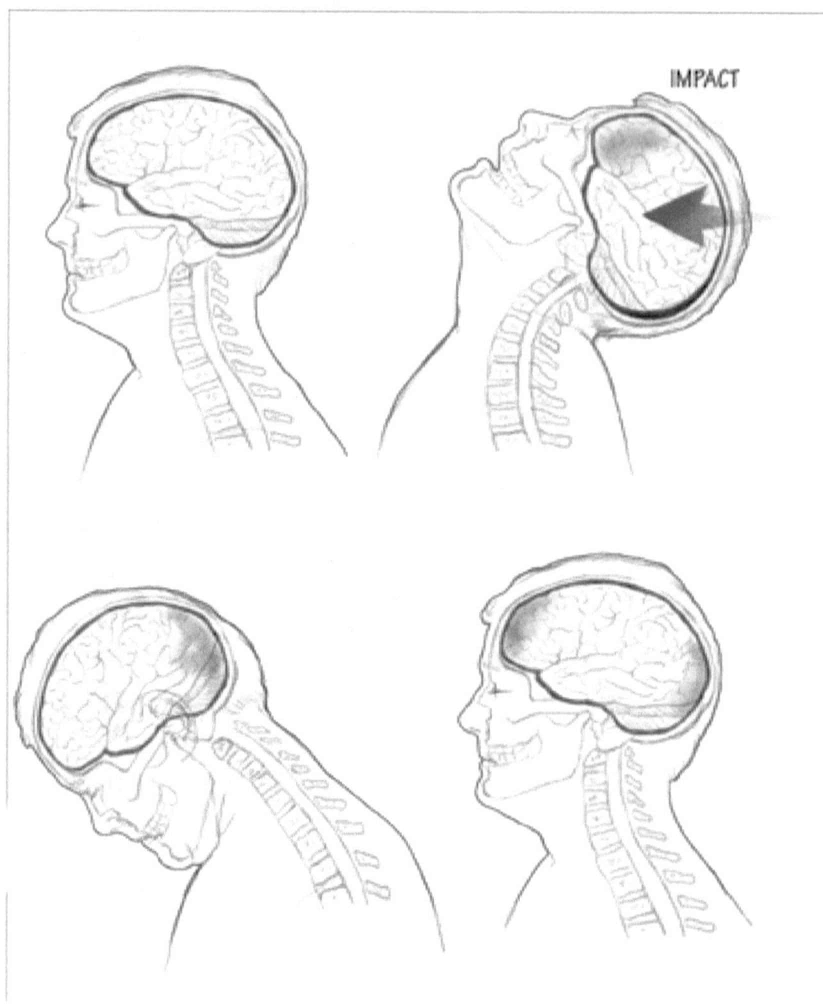

Figure 33. Areas of brain most frequently affected in post concussion syndrome.

There are also symptom complexes, which involve damage to multiple closely related structures resulting from trauma or injury, in the areas of the low back and pelvis. In the lumbar area there are discs that can become damaged. Some may be responsible for pain, and others not. Discs can also become degenerated, meaning they lose some height due to loss of water content. The damage to the facet joints and their nerves has been discussed, and damage to the lower lumbar facet joints is known to cause pain that radiates down to the buttocks and posterior knees but not below. This is a manifestation of damage to the facet joints, not radiculopathy, and it is a crucial distinction in making a correct diagnosis.

The pelvis is a ringlike structure made of cartilage and bone. In females, the pelvis is wider than in males to enable passage of a baby through the birth canal. There is also greater flexibility of the pubic symphysis and coccyx, which are the pelvic and tailbone portions of the birth canal, from hormones like progesterone that facilitate the birthing process. The pelvis attaches the lower extremities to the axial skeleton to allow for balance and locomotion. In cases of high-velocity trauma to the pelvis, the sacroiliac joints, which are posterior, can become damaged as well as the femoral and lateral femoral cutaneous nerves that pass near the inguinal (groin) area, which lie anteriorly and are fixed there due to fibrous tissue attachments. This situation predisposes these nerves to stretch injury in some cases of trauma.

In the neck area, the suprascapular nerve, which runs in the back of the shoulder, can also become stretched due to its ligamentous attachments to the scapula.

Stretch injury to nerves is a particularly vexing problem as it is difficult to diagnose, and nerves do not always fully recover. In many cases, identifying the damaged nerve and injecting the area around it with steroid and local anesthetic assists in making a diagnosis and treating the nerve injury. This is the only method currently available for diagnosing and treating a painful peripheral nerve, since there is no good physiologic test for the integrity of sensory nerves.

In this chapter, you have learned the following:

- About symptom complexes, which helps to explain the anatomic and physiologic reasons that injuries tend to cluster together.

- The development and role of peripheral nerve damage in chronic pain.

- The physics of outside forces working on our bodies to create injury.

- A main cause of headache following neck trauma.

Chapter 8

The Different Types of Arthritis

If you don't know what is causing your joint pain and stiffness, it is likely arthritis

The rapid evolution of medical technologies and treatments in recent years may allow for extreme longevity. As we become a longer-living, more overweight society, there are certain trade-offs that we as individuals and as a society have chosen.

When I think of all the patients I came in contact with as an intern in internal medicine in 1984, I am astounded by how far we have come in this short period of time. Back then, coronary angioplasty, which involves placing a dye into the arteries that supply blood and oxygen to the heart, was just coming into vogue. I remember learning about it from a cardiologist and immediately informed my aunt who had radiation to the breast many years earlier and at the time was suffering from chest pain due to the radiation damage to her coronary arteries. My aunt was one of the first to have coronary angioplasty in NYC, and it saved her from a difficult operation that was likely to be fraught with complications. *An important universal lesson in medicine is that despite our desire to do almost anything to help, less invasive procedures can be more targeted to the problem and produce much less tissue damage..* We have come a long way in delaying the effects of, and treating, a multitude of common heart problems in the last quarter century, and while people still die of cardiac problems, on average they die later with a better quality of life. The same can be said of diagnosis of and treatments for cancer, which has gone from being a death sentence in the past to a chronic illness to be managed in the present. Advances in heart disease and cancer treatments will only accelerate in the future, allowing us to live longer, better quality lives.

But at what cost?

There are two problems that have become tremendous challenges to our independence as we age. The first is mental illness and dementia, which is beyond the scope of our discussion. Putting that aside, the main concern that I have for our aging population is the cumulative effects of wear and tear on our joints over the course of a lifetime. This wear and tear on joints is commonly known as *osteoarthritis*, and it has spawned the multibillion-dollar industry of joint replacement. As we all know, prevention and early detection are much more valuable strategies than treatment. Once significant damage has been done, surgical intervention moves higher on the list of options. We must learn to take better care of our joints when we are young if we wish to experience a more pleasant aging process. This is a relatively new phenomenon, as a hundred years ago the average life span was about forty-five years, so for most, joint pain was not a major consideration. Today, with improved treatments for many previously fatal illnesses, we must concern ourselves with the proper maintenance and care of our joints. The simplest approach is to live a healthier lifestyle. There is no question that losing weight, cessation of smoking, using alcohol in moderation, and avoiding repetitive, dangerous, or risky physical activities will enhance joint health and well-being in most cases. There are also specific stretching therapies for the low back and neck that I will discuss in a later chapter.

There are also some unfortunate people who have either illness from birth or acquired illnesses that affect their joint health. Here are just a few that relate to the spine and can cause chronic pain.

Two structural conditions of the spine are spina bifida and spinal stenosis. Spina bifida (figure 34) is a congenital condition due to the failure of the neural tube to fuse at its far end. The results of this condition can run the gamut from paralysis and incontinence to no detectable problems. There can be degenerative joint pain from structural abnormalities, and this can be a difficult condition to treat depending on its severity.

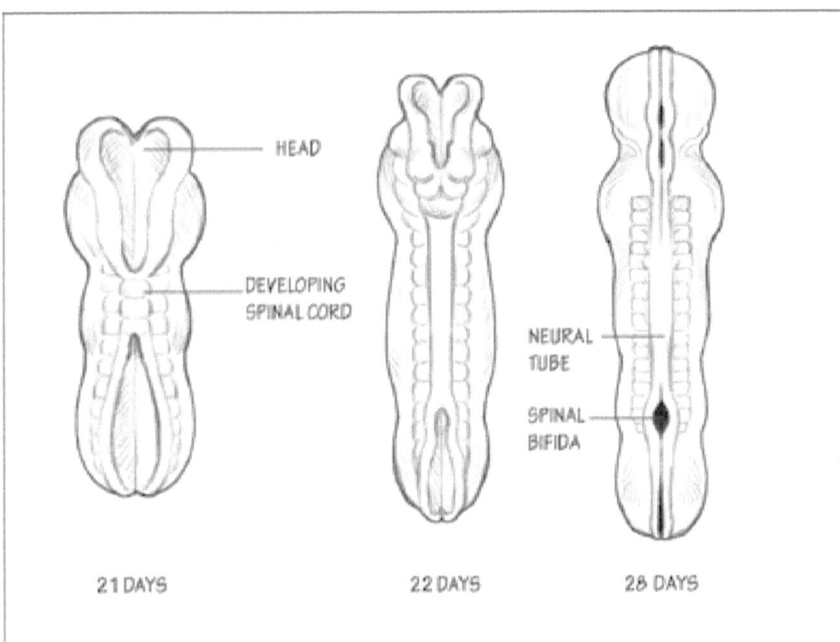

Figure 34. Neural tube defects in spina bifida.

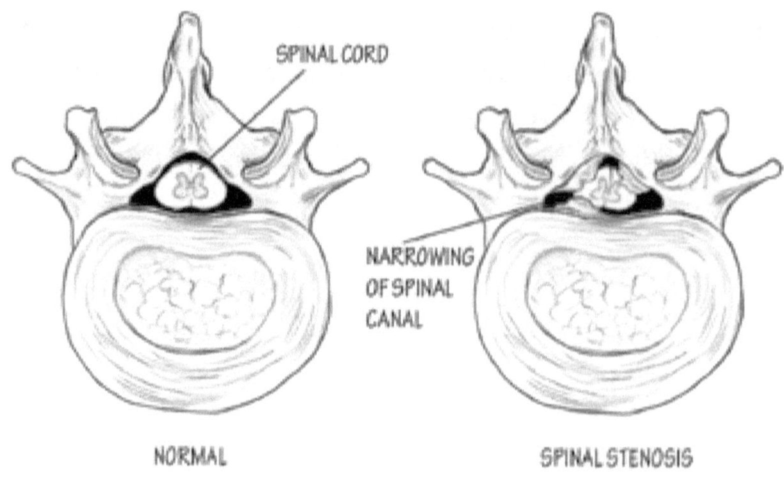

Figure 35. Compression of spine in spinal canal in advanced case of spinal stenosis.

Spinal stenosis (figure 35) can be either congenital or acquired. Some individuals are born with a spinal canal that has diminished dimensions, and the spinal cord can become compressed. In adults, arthritis can extend into the spinal canal, thus compromising the space available for the spinal cord. Spinal stenosis can cause numbness, weakness, tingling, and pain in the buttocks or extremities, but the hallmark of spinal stenosis in adults is pain in the lower extremities with even brief periods of ambulation or standing. This pain is not due to any circulatory abnormality and, as many forms of arthritis, is diminished with flexion of the spine and exacerbated by extension. (See figure 13.) For this reason, many patients with spinal stenosis tend to hunch forward. Sometimes epidural steroid injections help relieve the pain by decreasing inflammation, thus increasing the space in which the spinal cord can travel. In some cases, surgery will be necessary to decompress the spine. This will be discussed in the next chapter. I know that a patient is improving from epidural steroid injection when he or she is not slouching forward and is able to walk greater distances.

There are infectious causes for joint pain as well. Tuberculosis of the spine (Pott's disease) was a significant cause of neck/back pain in the past, due to infiltration of bacteria into bone and joint tissue. This may also occur in secondary syphilis. Another infectious illness that can cause intense low back pain is postpolio syndrome. Following the initial polio virus infection, there can be damage to and an imbalance of the musculature of the spine. This results in secondary asymmetrical wear and tear on the facet joints, causing a chronic pain syndrome after many years. These painful joints are successfully treated by injection of steroid medication.

There are metabolic disorders, such as Paget's disease of the spine, in which there is an imbalance between the buildup of bone and its reabsorption. Scoliosis, which causes abnormal curvature in the spine in growing adolescents, can cause abnormal forces to be generated in the facet joints, resulting in joint damage, and be responsible for chronic pain. Osteoporosis is a metabolic disorder in which bones become weak and brittle. Osteoporosis-related fractures commonly occur in the vertebral bodies, causing severe pain in women and the elderly (figure

36). Medications, a diet rich in calcium, and weight-bearing exercise can prevent bone loss and fractures.

Figure 36. Osteoporosis and painful vertebral body fracture.

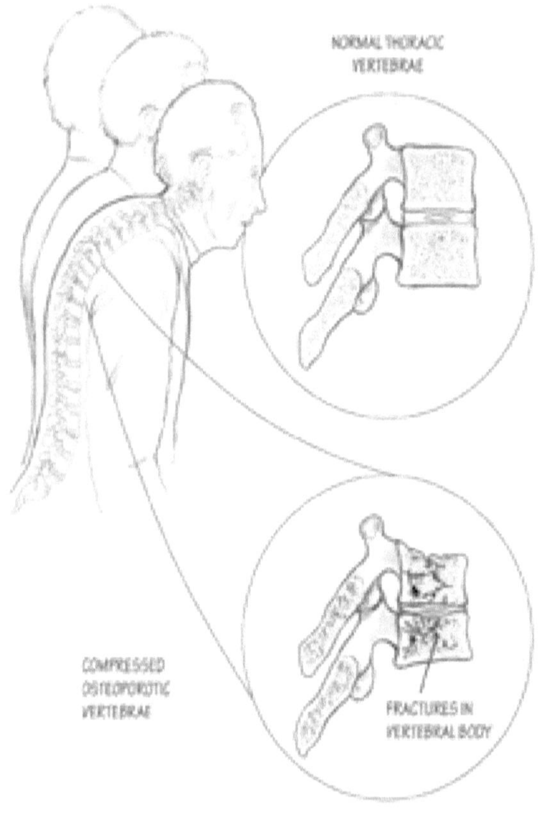

Cancer, whether primary or secondary, though a rare cause of back pain, can invade the bone and joints of the spine and place pressure upon sensitive nerve structures. Cancer that presents in this way can be undetected for many months before pressure is exerted on sensitive structures. It is important for patients to be sensitive to changes in their bodies, especially those that feel out of the ordinary relative to their experience. Cancer pain in the spine can also cause increased pain at night, due to the space-occupying effects of a cancerous lesion. These issues can only be explored after a thorough history and physical exam by a doctor and possibly with additional imaging tests.

Of all the causes of back and neck pain in the body, the most poorly characterized and understood are the autoimmune diseases. Autoimmune diseases are caused when the body's immune system, which under ordinary circumstances guards against foreign agents such as bacteria, viruses, fungi, and cancer cells, malfunctions and instead begins to attack the normal cells of the body. There are several autoimmune diseases that can contribute to chronic low back pain. The most prominent among these diseases is rheumatoid arthritis (RA). While RA is thought to occur in a symmetrical pattern in the joints of the hands and feet, it can also occur in the joints of the cervical and lumbar spines. Generally, arthritis is seen in the x-ray or MRI scan, and there may be antibodies called *rheumatoid factor* in the blood. There is generally a good deal of joint stiffness and pain, especially in advanced cases.

Another autoimmune cause of low back pain is known as *ankylosing spondylitis* (AS) (figure 37). AS has a strong genetic predisposition, and the most common symptom is back pain due to fusion of the sacroiliac joints and in severe cases of the discs as well. Symptoms can appear over many years. There are genetic and serologic tests that assist in diagnosis.

Inflammatory bowel diseases, such as Crohn's disease and ulcerative colitis, may also have an autoimmune component. In many cases, there are complaints of back pain in the areas of the lower lumbar facet joints and the sacroiliac joints for reasons that are unclear.

Sarcoidosis is an inflammatory disease that affects multiple organs but has a predilection for the lungs and lymph nodes. Joint pain can also occur in sarcoidosis, and the joints of the spine may become affected. *Systemic lupus erythematosus* is another systemic disease that can also affect joints of the lumbar and cervical spines.

It is not uncommon for the presenting symptom in some patients with autoimmune disorders to be experienced in the spine or pelvis. For patients with autoimmune or inflammatory diseases, I insist that their primary doctor should be a specialist who treats the particular type of disease that is causing the back pain symptoms. A rheumatologist is a specialist who treats these types of immunologic diseases with a variety of medications that modulate the immune system. In the case of inflammatory bowel disease, a gastroenterologist is the specialist who treats these illnesses with medications that suppress the immune system. Sarcoidosis is generally treated by pulmonologists.

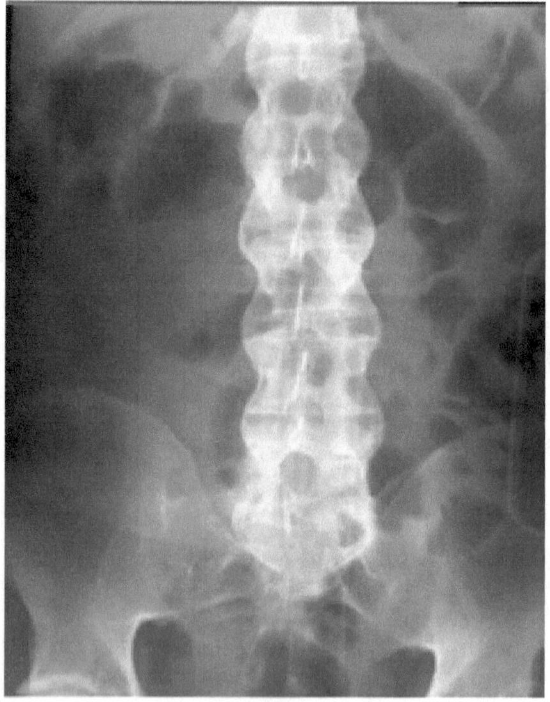

Figure 37. Ankylosing spondylitis. Case courtesy of Radio paedia.org, rID: 11189.

Once the inflammation in the body is under better control, there may be a role for the pain management specialist with medication management or joint injections. As in every other case of pain, making the proper diagnosis is of paramount importance, especially in cases of autoimmune diseases where delay in diagnosis can bring extensive joint destruction as well as other systemic manifestations.

Chronic pain is a symptom, not an illness; therefore, underlying causes for pain should always be sought.

In this chapter, you have learned the following:

- The importance of inflammation in the development of some cases of chronic pain

- Infection, cancer, metabolic, and immunologic diseases such as autoimmune disease are potent causes of inflammation

- Differential diagnosis for chronic pain should include causes of inflammation

Chapter 9

Situations in Which Surgery Is Unavoidable

Sometimes There Is No Choice

As you have progressed through this book, I am sure you realize that I am not the biggest proponent of spinal surgery. I do not want to leave you with the impression that spine surgery is never indicated; my only point is that we need be much more selective in our choice of candidates for surgery. The fact is that there are some cases in which spine surgery must be performed on an emergency basis. The failure to perform surgery in these cases may cause catastrophic disability or even death. In most of these cases, the need for surgery is quite obvious upon presentation of the patient in the emergency room.

In rare cases of high-velocity trauma, the vertebrae can fracture, resulting in compromise of the spinal cord. This is acute pain known as a burst fracture and occurs in the cervical, thoracic, or lumbar spines with associated numbness, weakness, and sometimes paralysis of an extremity. In order to minimize damage to the spinal cord, surgery must be performed rapidly in order to remove fragments of bone that are in the spinal canal as well as stabilization of the spine with plates and screws.

On any occasion in which the spinal cord becomes compressed from either tumor, blood clot, infection of bone or disc, or inflammation, and there is loss of motor (muscle) function or bowel or bladder tone, there is an urgent need for surgery in order to remove the tissue that is compressing the spine in order to rapidly restore neural function before permanent damage sets in (figure 38).

There are cases in which the ligaments holding the vertebral bodies in a stacked configuration, much like stackable building blocks, become lax (figure 39). This will result in the slippage of one vertebra relative to its neighbor, either forward or backward.

This condition is known as *spondylolisthesis,* and it generally does not represent a medical emergency. There is a slow progression of symptoms due to traction on the terminal branches of the spinal cord when this occurs in the lumbar spine. Symptoms include gait disturbance, forward leaning posture, numbness, tingling, weakness, and pain. There may be a slipping sensation with upright position. Flexion and extension x-rays are useful in determining the degree of slippage. If symptoms become significant, surgical stabilization is indicated.

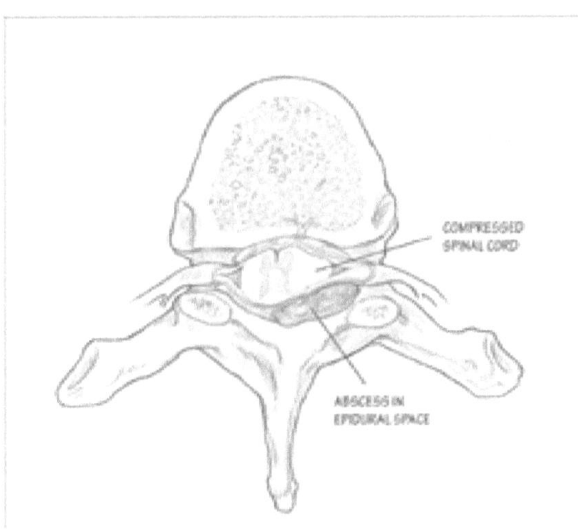

Figure 38. Spinal cord compression can be an emergency indication for surgery.

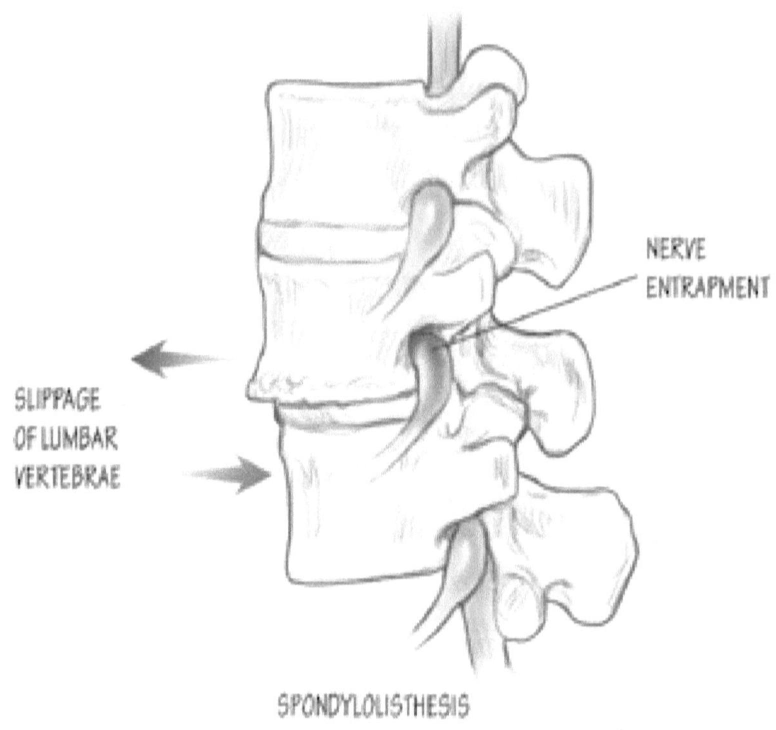

Figure 39. Spondylolisthesis. Laxity of spina ligaments results in slippage of vertebral bodies relative to each other.

Spinal stenosis in adults is a degenerative condition. The symptoms of spinal stenosis vary from patient to patient, but if it has become difficult to walk more than one block without back or leg pain and weakness as well as the onset of urinary incontinence, which would indicate significant compression of the terminal branches of the spinal cord, then surgery is indicated to decompress the lower spine. Failure to treat this condition surgically once symptoms begin to become significant will result in permanent weakness of the lower extremities and urinary incontinence over a period of years. In some cases of spinal stenosis, there is also instability of the spine, and spinal stabilization surgery (fusion) is also indicated.

Cauda equina syndrome (CES) is a rarely seen, serious neurological condition that requires immediate attention. CES occurs when the nerve fibers at the end of the spinal cord become compressed (figure 40), resulting in acute low back pain, tingling and numbness in the buttocks, bowel and bladder incontinence, loss of sexual function, loss of ankle reflexes, and weakness in the legs. Possible causes include acute herniated disc, infection, tumor, inflammation, hematoma, trauma, and spinal stenosis. There are no known risk factors for CES, and emergency surgical decompression is generally the only treatment option.

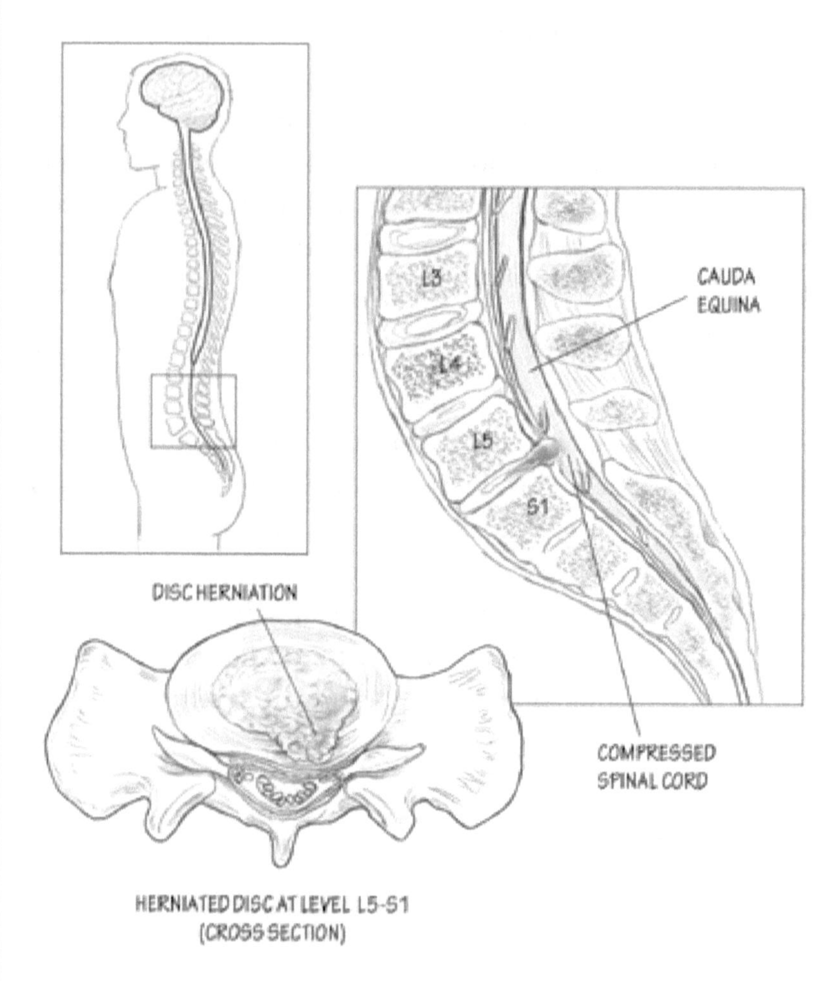

Figure 40. Cauda equina syndrome.

Vertebral body fractures from osteoporosis may need to be treated due to severe pain and loss of mobility, anorexia, and depression, especially in the elderly. Fractures of thoracic and lumbar vertebrae are most common and can occur with minimal exertion or even coughing or sneezing. Procedures such as vertebroplasty (figure 41) and kyphoplasty allow for the placement of bone cement into the vertebral body, thus stabilizing the fracture and in many cases significantly diminishing pain.

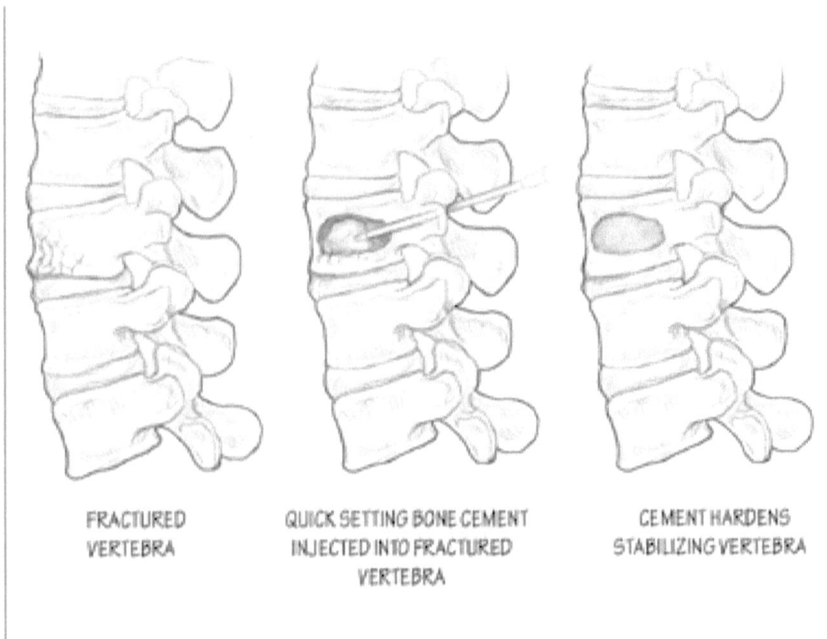

Figure 41. Vertebroplasty.

In this chapter, you have learned the following:

- That using the concepts in this book, neck and back surgery in many cases can be avoided, but there are always important exceptions.

- You must consult a physician specializing in the treatment of neck and back pain if pain persists for more than a few days, and there are cases when emergency care is indicated.

Chapter 10

Narcotic Analgesics and Other Pain-Relieving Medications

Damocles' Double-Edged Sword of Treatment

The story of Damocles is instructive for anyone who thinks that medical therapy is without its perils. The story goes that Dionysius, the tyrant of Syracuse, had a courtier named Damocles, who was a professional flatterer who lay around the king's opulent feasts, complimenting him effusively. Once he commented how wonderful it would be to be the king. Dionysius responded that Damocles could sit on his throne, which was well stocked with all sorts of creature comforts. There was just one catch. Dionysius placed a sword suspended only by a single horsehair above the throne, and when Damocles noticed the precarious position of the sword, he promptly abdicated the throne.

In this life, there are no free rides. Something that seems to be a very good idea can also have many undesirable features. This, in essence, is the problem and the controversy that swirls around the medicines we use to treat painful conditions. The most difficult and challenging aspects of working with people in chronic pain is first to get the correct or proper diagnosis. The premise of this book is that there are many diagnostic possibilities in chronic pain patients that are not considered frequently enough. After making a diagnosis, the next challenge is to formulate a treatment plan. In many cases, medications are prescribed to try to diminish the pain; the type of medication prescribed will be geared to what the physician has identified as the mechanism of pain.

For instance, if the pain is inflammatory and minor and involving a ligament or muscle, I may prescribe aspirin, Tylenol, or ibuprofen; for moderate pain, codeine, tramadol, or hydrocodone. If there is only nerve pain or headache from nerve irritation, antiseizure medications such as pregabalin, gabapentin, or topiramate are useful. Some physicians will treat pain and depression with antidepressants such as Elavil, Pamelor, or Cymbalta. If there is a component of muscle spasm, then antispasmodics such as Flexeril, Soma, or Tizanidine are used. If there is a discrete area of inflammation in a muscle, tendon, or ligament, a topical anti-inflammatory gel, such as Voltaren Gel or Lidoderm, or Flector patches are very helpful.

There are many other medicines, patches, and rubs available for the consumer, but the basic premise of the pharmacology of pain relief is to either reduce spasm and inflammation or to modulate the peripheral nervous system so that painful impulses have to work harder to propagate their message, or to alter the central nervous system so that pain-relieving chemicals that mimic the ones we naturally have in our brain (endorphins) are released in the synapses or junctions of nerves. The problem with all these medications is that they are relatively nonspecific treatments for problems that are difficult to identify. If we could hone down on the mechanisms of pain, not only on a basic science, molecular level but also by looking at the larger picture of nerve tissue damage and injury, new solutions may emerge.

In my specialty, there is the perfect storm of patients who are suffering and demanding that doctors do something to help them ("Isn't that why you became a doctor?"), the confounding human anatomic and physiologic relationships that are confusing as to the origin of the pain, the frustration of the medical community with patients who do not get better ("I don't understand. I did everything to help him, and he is still complaining. Is there something wrong with him? Should I send him to a therapist?"), and the imperfect medications that definitely help to relieve symptoms but offer very little in the way of cure. Worse than that, the gold standard of pain relief, the narcotics or opioids, can cause both physiological and psychological dependence. If that is not bad enough, in recent years the incidence of narcotic overdose has multiplied fourfold in the United States. There were approximately seventeen thousand deaths from prescription narcotic overdose in 2012 in the United States.[17] By comparison, about sixteen thousand die per year from complications of Tylenol, aspirin, and ibuprofen; it is not only the narcotic analgesics that are a problem![18]

In the opinion of many doctors, chronic pain should be treated as a disease, such as hypertension or diabetes, and therefore patients should not be left in severe pain for days and hours on end because of the potential damage to the circulatory system, heart and brain, and other tissues from prolonged periods of stress. This seems very reasonable until you consider the other side. There are a small but significant number of chronic pain patients that become addicted to narcotic analgesics in the course of treatment (1–20 percent). This does not mean that they are bad people but rather that they can experience a euphoric effect from using and abusing narcotics, and due to genetic factors, they begin to seek these drugs. These patients are at extra risk when prescribed these powerful painkillers. The temptation to feel good can be so great that patients add other nonprescribed drugs to their regimen, such as alcohol, heroin, fentanyl, and cocaine, in order to prolong the high. Fortunately, this is not the case for the majority of chronic pain patients.

These addicts deserve our compassion and understanding, because if not for having been injured or having pain following surgery, these vulnerable

---

17   CDC WONDER online database, 2012.
18   NSAIDs, Consumer Health Choices, consumerhealthchoices.org, 2012/02.

individuals would never have been exposed to those powerful chemicals that cause the physical and psychological effects. I am not saying that these people are victims, just that we should try to understand how they became addicted to opiates. There are also some nefarious individuals who pretend to have chronic pain so that they can have access to narcotics from their doctors. I have no compassion for these people, because they either use the narcotics to become high or they sell them on the street for profit. This behavior causes great suspicion about the utility and efficacy of these medications among physicians, law enforcement, and lay people and brings about the restriction of these powerful medications to the very people who need them the most. In my opinion, these people should have to attend drug rehabilitation programs if applicable and be prosecuted to the full extent of the law for their callous disregard of true pain sufferers and members of the community. It is also very wrong for chronic pain patients to share a few of their pills with friends, family, and coworkers. Having a bottle of pills in no way makes you a healer.

There are physical consequences of narcotic usage. Acutely, there is the risk of respiratory depression, the cessation of the drive to breathe by the attachment of narcotics to certain receptors in the brain. This is an especially important consideration in people with lung or liver disease as well as patients who have taken too much narcotics (overdose). In recent times, police have become equipped with the narcotic reversal agent Narcan, which is a necessary but sad commentary on the degree of drug misuse and abuse in our society. Other effects of narcotics can be nausea, vomiting, constipation, and diminished testosterone, causing decreased libido. There is also the problem of withdrawal or physical dependence. Discontinuing narcotics suddenly, for some patients, will cause gastrointestinal upset, feelings of discomfort and irritability, sweating, and flu-like symptoms. Dependence is a physical phenomenon, while addiction is a psychological one.

There is also a tendency for doctors who do not want to be bothered by patient complaints to prescribe benzodiazepines (minor tranquilizers/ anxiety relievers) such as valium, Xanax, or trazodone. These medications are used to relax the muscles, and some studies have found these medications to be more addictive than the narcotics. These medications relax your mind as well as your body so that cares and unpleasant memories melt away. These medications should never be used for the long term. Anxiety should be dealt with in the context of psychological therapy. Muscle relaxants are available that do not interfere with alertness and cognition. The most problematic drug interactions occur when these anxiolytics are taken together with narcotics, which will definitely cause drowsiness, sleepiness, and altered cognition. This combination is especially dangerous with driving or operating heavy machinery. I try to avoid prescribing anxiolytics because treatment of anxiety is out of the scope of pain medicine. Patients must also remember not to drink alcohol while taking pain medications for similar reasons. Big pharma is constantly on the search for pain-relieving medications that are more targeted and that do not have the problems associated with narcotic analgesics.

We as a society need to step back and try to sort through all the facts and rationally create rules that will not allow the unfettered distribution of prescription narcotics to nonchronic pain patients while allowing true patients not to be restricted from the medications they so desperately may need in order to perform simple activities of daily living. It is one of the challenges of pain management doctors to adjust these medications so that there is a balance between the pain-relieving properties of narcotics, versus their side effects and also the potential for abuse and diversion. This is a worthy goal that is difficult to achieve.

Physicians generally prescribe these medications only after a proper history and physical exam. It is no small matter to begin treatment of a patient on these medications, because they must be monitored for behavioral changes throughout the course of therapy. It is also useful to discuss with the patient an exit strategy. How long will the narcotic be tried and what options are there to decrease or suspend opiate usage? I have found that patients who are not compliant with the treatment plan that I give them at the initial consultation do not handle their medications properly. It makes sense that someone who only wants to take the narcotics on their own terms really does not wish to get better. We try very hard to separate the real patients from the imposters with random urine tests and prescription monitoring reports, but even these methods are not infallible, and some false patients do get access to narcotics (until they are caught).

There will be a time in the future when the mechanisms of chronic pain will become more fully clarified, and the current pain medications will become obsolete. Until that time, I would hope that as a society we are able to show compassion and humanity toward those whose lives are filled with pain and suffering. In cases where it is appropriate, to treat patients with suboptimal amounts of pain medications is tantamount to not treating them at all. There may be some unintended consequences of *undertreating* patients. From the early 1990s when pain was to be measured as the fifth vital sign,[19] we have seen multiple cases of abuse and misuse of these powerful medications. Now the pendulum has swung to the other extreme with legitimate pain patients unable to find a doctor willing to treat them with opiates. This is all understandable; there are powerful arguments to be made on both sides. Clearly a more neutral position will benefit the greatest number of patients. Physicians working together with law enforcement would help to curtail improper narcotic use to the greatest degree. Most importantly, patients need to take responsibility for their treatments, to make their best effort to live with less pain by nonpharmacologic means, and to advocate to the regulatory agencies for themselves.

I did not choose to specialize in pain management because I had an interest in law enforcement; I would prefer to think the best of my patients. Unfortunately, some bad experiences have soured most pain-management specialists, and the onus from regulatory and licensing bureaus is on us to be vigilant. I still try to give patients the benefit of the doubt because I believe everyone should have a chance to live with less pain, but it is very demoralizing to find patients who are not honest and are not using their medications properly. In the future, chronic pain patients will need to

---

19   Pain as the Fifth Vital Sign, NCBI, www.ncbi.nlm.gov.

relinquish some of their privacy rights in order to secure their medications and to ensure that opiate medications are not abused or misused.

In this chapter, you have learned the following:

- The pit falls of managing chronic pain with narcotics.

- How a new paradigm for chronic pain presented in this book can lead to the proper diagnosis and treatment of pain and can mitigate the need for narcotics as a long- term treatment.

Chapter 11

Non pharmacological Therapies That May Be Helpful

"First Do No Harm"

From the outset, it should be clear that most cases of neck/LBP are amenable to some form of noninvasive treatment. It is the rare patient who needs neck/back surgery. If someone is pushing you to have spinal surgery from the first encounter, unless it is one of the surgical urgencies or emergencies mentioned in Chapter 9, you should bolt out of that office as soon as you can. Even if you are offered a "minimally invasive technique," if there is no emergency, you should try these nonpharmacological therapies first.

Since this book features the mind-body connection prominently, I feel that it is always worth the effort to try relaxation techniques, such as meditation or breathing exercises or yoga. There is a large component of the pain experience that is processed in the brain, and there are also emotional and cognitive factors that play a significant role. Ignoring the role that perception, feelings, and emotions play will result in seeking help through medications and surgery, which should be your last options, not the first. Obviously, in an acute situation, taking some aspirin or ibuprofen or muscle relaxant will be helpful, but for chronic pain, some form of psychological technique should be employed regularly. These techniques may not eliminate chronic pain, but they help to make pain more tolerable.

Many people get relief from chiropractic manipulation. The relief is good and usually lasts for several days, necessitating multiple office visits. It makes sense why manipulation helps. If much of the pain relates to the joints of the spine, then moving the joints will afford some relief possibly by temporarily interrupting the transmission of painful sensations from the facet joints to the spine. Many have found chiropractic care helpful and noninvasive for neck/back pain.

Physical therapy is also useful for the majority of patients and allows for strengthening and conditioning of core muscles that support the axial skeleton as well as gentle stretching of tendons and ligaments. Some patients cannot perform the activities in physical therapy due to their pain. These patients have likely sustained either nerve injury or injury to the facet joints, which are painful with motion due to the nature of these conditions. These patients will improve with time, but the nerve injury and damage to facet joints need to be addressed with nerve blocks prior to any physical therapy, in order to allow the patient to be more comfortable in the course of treatment.

Stretching of tendons and ligaments is very important for all of us as we age. As tissues in the body contain less water, they become less elastic; this is part of the normal aging process. We must all be vigilant as we get older to stretch prior to any exertion or physical activity. The joints of the spine tend to become stiff at night since we are not moving to the same degree as during the daytime, and our bodies are in a recumbent position, allowing for the accumulation of a small amount of fluid in the joints. The cervical and lumbar spines should be stretched at night and in the mornings in order to diminish stiffness and pain (figures 42 and 43).

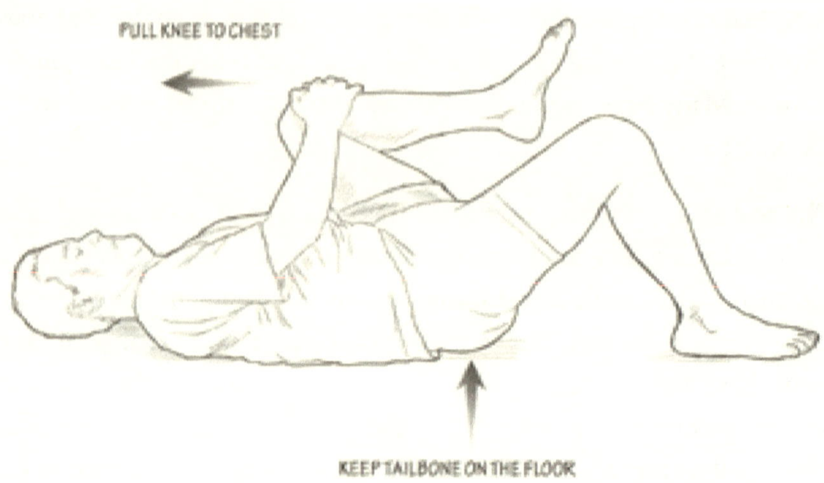

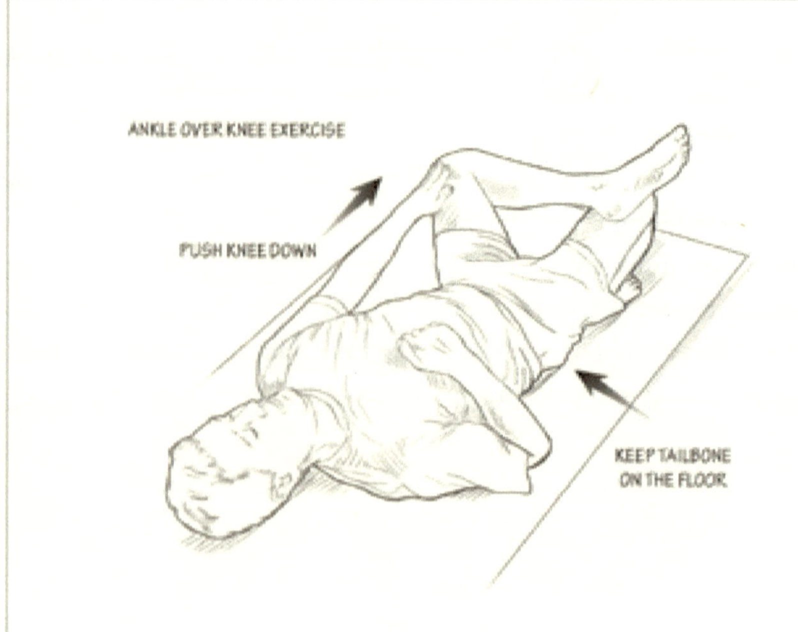

Figures 42 and 43. Stretching exercises.

Many chronic low back pain sufferers have benefitted from the McKenzie Method, which utilizes stretching techniques that patients can perform at home to treat chronic musculoskeletal injury (www.mckenzieinstituteusa.org).

Swimming is an excellent way to get exercise if you have neck or back pain. The buoyancy of the water allows for greater freedom of motion of joints throughout the body. Patients who swim two to three times a week are able to keep muscles in better condition and also have a greater sense of well-being from the exercises that they are able to do in the water. The Arthritis Foundation (www. arthritis.org) is an excellent resource for anyone looking for water exercise. It really works!

Acupuncture is another therapeutic option. This Eastern medicine technique involves placing very small, thin needles into the body at specific acupuncture points along lines called *meridians*. Acupuncture is used to treat a variety of painful conditions. It is not clear what the mechanism of action for pain relief is, and it is also not clear from scientific studies whether this is an effective treatment for chronic pain.

Many patients over the years have had success using inversion tables (figure 44). Inversion tables are similar to the old traction apparatus in terms of the way the spine is gently distracted (pulled apart). Inversion tables use gravity to do the work of stretching and separating the ligaments and vertebrae. In that sense, this treatment is similar to traction or chiropractic manipulation but can be performed at home.

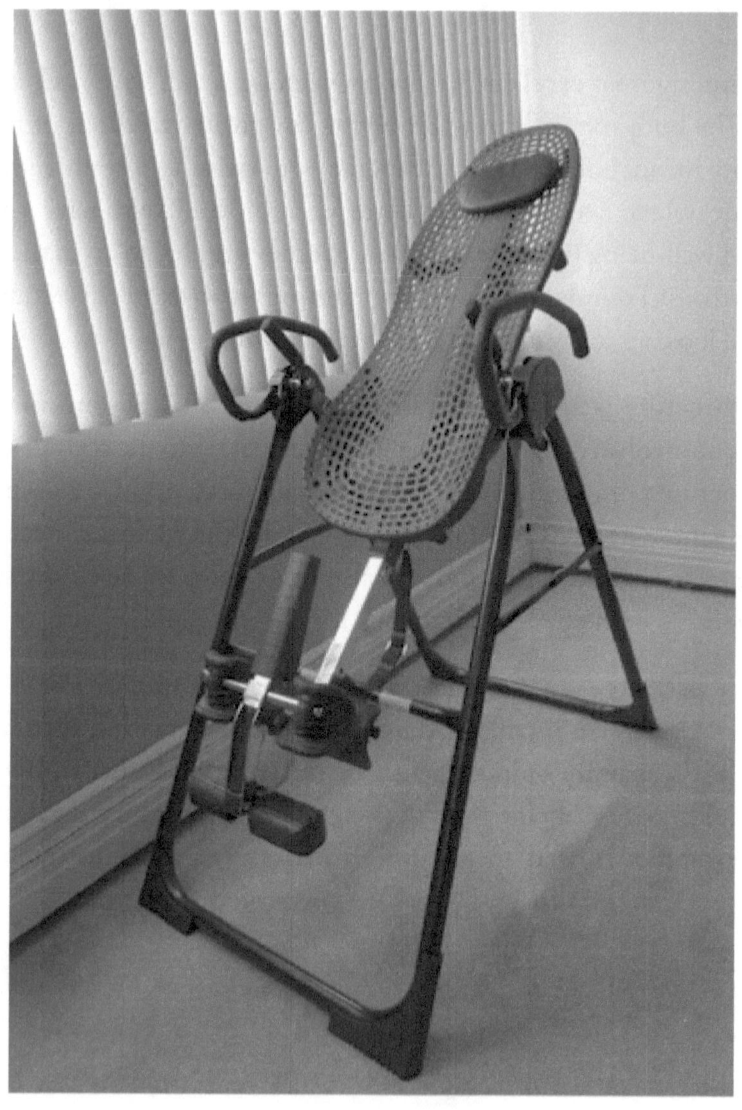

Figure 44- Inversion table By Giorgostr via Wikimedia Commons

Massage helps some patients symptomatically by helping to release muscle spasm. It is always advantageous to know what types of treatments are helpful to relieve your pain and also to be able to do some simple therapies at home. Your spine needs several minutes a day of preventative maintenance as you age and also as you begin to increase your activity level, in order to avoid chronic neck/back pain.

Neuromodulation involves using electrical stimulation to provide pain relief.

TENS or transcutaneous electrical nerve stimulation simply involves placing electrodes over the spinal levels experiencing pain and pulsing electrical energy via a small generator that can be worn on the belt. In my experience, TENS works particularly well for painful vertebral body fractures. It has been used to treat degenerative disc disease and arthritis as well.

Spinal cord stimulation (figure45) requires the implantation of an internal electrode and generator under anesthesia. SCS is primarily used to treat scar tissue build up that sometimes results from back surgery called *epidural fibrosis*. It may also be used to treat neuropathic (nerve-related) pain in the extremities, called *chronic regional pain syndrome*.

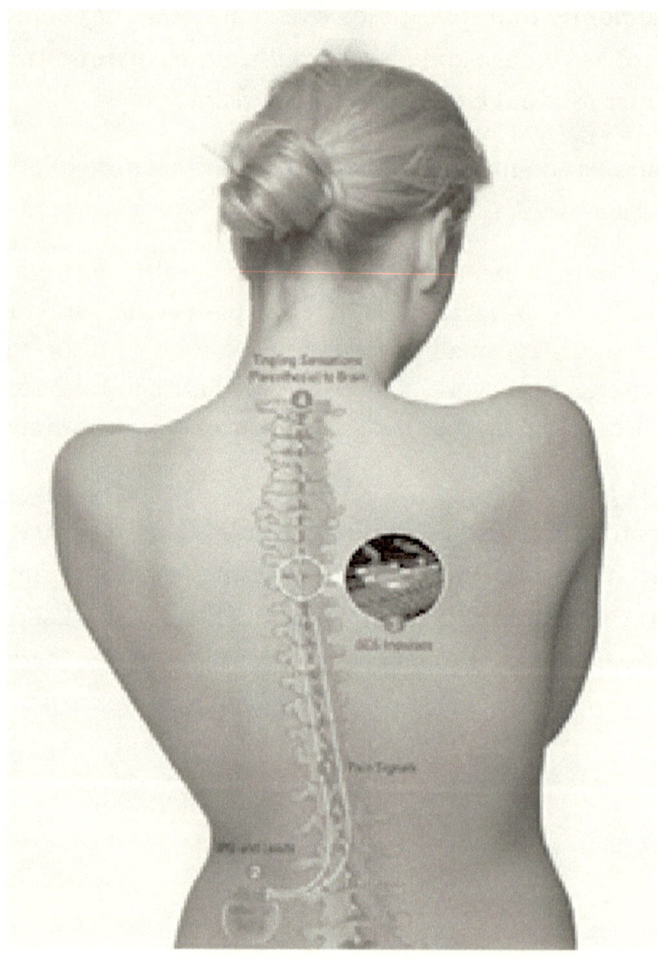

Figure 45. Spinal cord stimulator.

In this chapter, you have learned the following:

- About alternative therapies for treatment of chronic pain.

- That stretching is an essential strategy for diminishing pain or injury as we age due to the decreasing water content of our tissues.

- There are many ways that patients can take control of their own pain.

Chapter 12

Hope for the Future, Paths for Healing

To Boldly Persevere Until the Solution Arrives

If my investments are any indication of my ability to predict future events and trends, then I have no business writing about the future. Rather than prognosticate, however, it is fairly easy to see some of the areas that need further exploration in the future and to suggest ways that those goals can be attained.

It is very easy to declare a war on drugs but a much more complicated feat to declare a war on chronic pain. The pages of history generally record events from the perspective of the victors. Who will be the winners and losers in this war? Not many people today are aware of the challenges of their ancestors of four or five generations ago. Will our grandchildren suffer from pain in the same fashion that we experience it, or will there be more effective diagnostic tests and treatments? We are most familiar with our world in the present, but the most interesting individuals are the ones who can look beyond the status quo, identify problems that need correction, and find innovative solutions. How we handle heart disease and cancer has steadily evolved over the past twenty five years because clinicians and patients were not satisfied with the results. Now I believe it is time for the same type of attention to be paid to people suffering daily with chronic pain.

There is one characteristic of pain management as a specialty that sets it apart from every other medical specialty. It is clear that pain is a highly subjective experience that is difficult for the observer to measure or diagnose. In almost all other areas of medicine, except psychiatry, there are useful, verifiable, and accepted tests that help isolate and define trauma, illness, or disease. Since acute pain is a symptom and not a disease, medical testing is useful in the search for diagnostic possibilities. Once pain has become chronic, it moves into the realm of chronic illness, with few if any reliable objective features. I have given several explanations as to why this may be so. There is always a fine balance between the central and peripheral nervous systems, with information and messages constantly and rapidly being shared between the spinal cord, brain, and outside environment.

For all these reasons, patients with chronic pain and the doctors who treat them are always suspected of improper use and prescription, respectively, of pain-relieving medications. In an ideal world, the process of measuring and gauging pain would be objectified to the extent that chronic pain could be quantified. In a best-case scenario, tissue damage could be demonstrated. This certainly goes against the opinion of those who say that chronic pain is a mind-body experience that does not have any organic (physical) basis. We no longer attribute that which we do not understand and cannot see to the gods, or supernatural factors, or magic, or even to our imagination or our response to stress. All these reasons are possible, but we must also ask, as we become more sophisticated, what are the possibilities and the probabilities of back pain being exclusively in the province of the mind-body or subjective-spiritual realm?

For many years, gastric ulcers were thought to be induced by stress. Stress and acid production in the stomach appeared to be the main causes of gastric ulcers, and many patients had gastric surgery to reconfigure their stomach and its innervation so that further damage to the stomach could be averted. About thirty years ago, it was found that there is a bacterium, *H. pylori*, that can thrive in the acidic environment of the stomach (something thought not possible), and treatment for the bacterial infection and for the buildup of acid has virtually eliminated the need for surgery for gastric ulcers. Here is an example of an illness that for many years was thought to have a psychosomatic basis and has been shown to be caused, in many cases, by infection. Medical knowledge is always evolving, and just because we do not yet understand the cause of a disease or illness is not reason to condemn the patient.

Sadly, we are not able to measure the degree of pain a patient is experiencing. Because of that fact, we are not able to distinguish chronic pain patients from the posers who only want pain medications. There are numerous problems associated with prescription of narcotic analgesics. There have been attempts to measure pain experimentally by looking at changes in the cortex of the brain using functional MRI and PET imaging when pain has been induced. Unfortunately, these efforts have not yielded the desired results, and it is not cost effective to place every chronic pain patient in an MRI or PET scanner to measure pain levels. I am not a researcher, but it seems to me that if only the peripheral sensory mechanism is damaged, looking at the brain to measure pain is like looking at the central processing unit of a computer to find a malfunction that actually exists in the keyboard or mouse. Once information has gone from the spine to the brain, it is highly processed with multiple inputs and chemical reactions so that it no longer resembles the original input.

It might be worthwhile to attempt to measure pain at the affected spinal levels in a fashion similar to the way noise-cancelling technology works. In theory, we should be able to gauge painful impulses at the level they enter the spine by slowly increasing an *external* painful stimulus such as heat or electricity to such a point that the sensory experience from chronic pain is overwhelmed by the externally applied painful stimulus. The amount of stimulus (current or heat) can be quantified and measured on a scale, theoretically. If this technique provides useful information, it could be performed quite rapidly and inexpensively.

Once we are able to quantify and measure pain, the next step would be to actually identify damage to the peripheral nerves that have been stretched or compressed from trauma or inflammation. I think that the field of molecular imaging for pain is the hope for the future. Many researchers prefer to image the brain to search for causes of pain, but if, in many cases pain is due to peripheral nerve injury, then imaging of the brain represents the final product of all the inputs in the body that have contributed to the experience of pain. This, in theory, should be much more complicated to measure and interpret than assess the actual site of damage that incites the barrage of stimuli that are processed in the brain.

Proteins that are formed in the areas of damaged nerves have been identified. Our genetic system turns on genes in the cell bodies and certain specialized proteins that are expressed only when nerves are damaged. These new proteins can be radiolabeled so that they are visible to a PET scanner or source of ultraviolet light, thus identifying the area of nerve damage. This type of objective test is not available today, but if it were possible to image damaged nerves, areas of compression could be relieved, and areas of transection or severe damage could be resected and reconnected. Today this concept is science fiction, but I do believe that we will be able to image inflamed or damaged nerves in several years. This will revolutionize the field of pain management in the same way the discovery of *H. Pylori* revolutionized treatment of gastric ulcers. This will also remove many chronic pain patients from the realm of pure psychological illness to a more organic diagnosis, when appropriate. If this test is very sensitive, it will enable us to distinguish the true pain patients from the drug seekers.

In terms of medications and therapies, because of the epidemic of drug abuse, which occurs frequently in the setting of chronic pain management, there is a move by drug developers to create drugs that relieve pain without the psychological or physiological cravings. In recent years there has been tremendous interest in regenerative therapies such as stem cells and nerve growth factor which may allow more rapid and complete restoration of damaged peripheral nerves, cartilage in joints, and disc material which has become degenerated and painful. In fact, there is now a company that claims to produce reduction of low back pain with 87% efficacy by using stem cells. By restoring normal architecture in peripheral nerves, genes that are activated by nerve damage and areas of the brain that are involved in the pain experience could become quiescent. Turning off the activated central nervous system is an essential goal for treating any chronic pain sufferer.

The issue of misuse and abuse of narcotic analgesics is a troubling development that has increased along with the stated goal of diminishing the suffering of chronic pain patients. It is incumbent upon every prescriber of opiates to spend time with the patient to explain strategies for successful dosing. It is not sufficient just to give a patient powerful painkillers; they must also know what times and intervals medications should be used, for what purposes (narcotic analgesics are not a treatment for anxiety), and what the goals of treatment are. They should also be familiar with adverse effects and side effects. Most important, patients need to understand that increased pain is an indication of increased inflammation. Rather than taking extra pills, the escalation of pain is an indication for reevaluation, and a nerve block or joint injection will usually quell the pain. It is interesting to note that the escalation of narcotic dosage rarely makes a difference in the intensity of pain or ability to increase activity levels.

Today there are tremendous constraints on the prescription of pain medications. I understand that there are many patients with chronic non cancer pain who are unable to find a doctor who will treat their pain adequately with opiates. In my experience, some patients have a lax attitude toward their pain medications and do not handle them properly. I have refused to prescribe narcotics to patients with roommates or small children until they have purchased a safe to protect their medications at home. At this time, with computers so pervasive in society, there will likely come a time that chronic pain patients will have to purchase a small drug-dispensing machine for the home, connected to the Internet, so that the patterns of narcotic use can be reviewed by their specialist. If medications are abused or misused, the drug-dispensing machine will record aberrant patterns of use. Obviously, this machine must be inexpensive to own, determine whether it has been properly loaded, be able to count pills, distribute pills one at a time, and record and transmit relevant information. Under these circumstances, abuse and misuse of narcotic analgesics could be significantly curtailed. The proper use and restriction of these powerful medications is in the interest of every member of our society.

Conclusion

Treating chronic pain requires tremendous teamwork involving patients, family, doctors, pharmacists, and physical and psychological therapists. Patients should not be blamed for their chronic pain anymore than crime victims should bear blame for their circumstances.

I have always enjoyed educating my patients about their pain. In many cases, they are relieved to have an understanding of the nature of their problem. Many patients live with pain for *years* without any idea of why they are suffering. I have been fortunate to have been able to help patients understand the mechanism and causes of their pain because of my unique perspective. Unfortunately, so much chronic pain is treated inadequately for various reasons. The improper treatment of pain is responsible for wasting hundreds of millions of dollars and needless prolonged suffering annually, because there are not standard treatment regimens for pain that has become chronic. This lack of proper diagnosis and treatment, in many cases of chronic pain, lends an air of despair and helplessness to the doctor-patient relationship. These feelings may contribute to the over-prescription of narcotic analgesics. I hope that you are now aware of what happens to your body with trauma or arthritis, which types of treatment will be helpful, and which ones to avoid. If I have given you just this, then you have gained much.

About the Author

Jordan Fersel, MD, is a board-certified, pain-management fellowship-trained physician who earned a BA in biology from Queens College and an MD degree from Mount Sinai School of Medicine. He has been director of Pain Management Services at Trinitas Medical Center Oncology Unit for several years. Dr. Fersel and his wife, Esty, divide their time between Philadelphia and West Orange, New Jersey.

Index

A

B

C

misuse (of narcotics) 3, 106, 108, 122, 123

molecular imaging, as hope for future 121

motor (locomotive) output 22

motor vehicle accident (MVA) 9, 67

MRIs 12, 15, 46

multiple sensors 32

muscle 63

Muscle relaxants 107

muscle spasm XIII, 8, 45, 83, 104, 115

myelogram 10

N

Narcan 106

narcotic analgesics 3, 4, 105, 107, 120, 122, 123, 125

needles, in HANDS acronym 20

nerve block 53, 122

nerve compression 68, 69

nerve entrapment, 98

nerve growth factor, 121-122

nerve injury 45, 49, 61, 62, 68, 71, 78, 80, 81, 83, 85, 111, 121

nerve root 11, 14, 30, 31, 35, 37, 41, 42, 62, 71, 74, 77

nerves

    afferent (sensory) nerves 30, 62
    autonomic nerves 33
    damaged (severed) nerve reconstitution, 66-67
    efferent (motor or other response to stimulus) nerves, 30, 62
    femoral nerve, 60, 77
    first order nerves, 64
    lateral femoral cutaneous nerve, 6, 60, 68, 77
    peripheral nerves, 45,49, 66, 67 77, 78, 121, 122
    possible function of ones found on surface of vertebrae and disc, 34
    radial nerve, 70
    sensory nerves, 64
    sinuvertebral nerve, 29, 30, 32, 33, 34, 35
    somatic nerves, 30, 35
    spinal nerve, 31f, 32f
    suprascapular nerve, 85
    ulnar nerve, 70f

nervous system. *See also* autonomic nervous system; central nervous system (CNS); peripheral nervous system
    as biological system, 22
    as body's electrical system, 22
    functions of, XV
    relationship between autonomic and somatic nervous systems, 29f
    neural tube defects, 89f
    neuritis, 68
    neuroaugmentation, 20
    neuromodulation, 115
    neuromuscular disorders, diagnosis of, 49
    neuropathy, 35, 45, 68,
    Newton, Isaac, 80

noise-cancelling technology 120

noninvasive treatment 110

nonpharmacological therapies 110

nucleus pulposus 14, 35

numbness 39, 56, 68, 69, 70, 71, 72, 91, 96, 97, 99

O

ontogeny recapitulates phylogeny 21